Simon & Schuster

NEW YORK   LONDON   TORONTO   SYDNEY   SINGAPORE

Reinventing Yourself

❧ with ❧

The Duchess of York

INSPIRING STORIES
AND STRATEGIES FOR
CHANGING YOUR WEIGHT
AND YOUR LIFE

Sarah, The Duchess of York
and Weight Watchers

A Word About Weight Watchers

Since 1963, Weight Watchers has grown from a handful of people to millions of enrollments annually. Today, Weight Watchers is recognized as the leading name in safe and sensible weight control. Weight Watchers members form diverse groups, from youths to senior citizens, attending meetings virtually around the globe. Weight-loss and weight-management results vary by individual but we recommend that you attend Weight Watchers meetings, follow the Weight Watchers food plan and participate in regular physical activity. For the Weight Watchers meeting nearest you, call 1-800-651-6000. Also, visit us at our Web site, www.weightwatchers.com.

WEIGHT WATCHERS PUBLISHING GROUP
CREATIVE & EDITORIAL DIRECTOR: NANCY GAGLIARDI
EDITORIAL ASSISTANT: JENNY LABOY-BRACE
WRITER: STACEY COLINO, M.S.

SIMON & SCHUSTER
Rockefeller Center, 1230 Avenue of the Americas,
New York, NY 10020

SIMON & SCHUSTER and colophon are registered trademarks of
Simon & Schuster, Inc.

Designed by Jill Weber
Permissions acknowledgments appear on page 223.
Manufactured in the United States of America
1   3   5   7   9   10   8   6   4   2

ISBN 0-7432-1330-0

Contents

Reinventing Yourself with The Duchess of York

Introduction

*P*eople often ask me whether I'd rewrite my own history if I could. It's an intriguing thought. Certainly there were dark periods in my life when I would have welcomed the chance to be someone else. Today I feel much differently, though, because I've learned so much from my past; looking back, even the difficult times served a purpose in shaping the stronger and more confident person I've become. I am who I am because of my life, not despite it.

It's fitting that my personal crest reads *Ex adversis felicitas crescit,* which loosely translated from Latin could mean "out of adversity comes happiness." When my world unraveled spectacularly a while ago I thought my life was over. I felt overwhelmed by insurmountable obstacles, and my out-of-control weight problem was the most obvious symptom of a much deeper emotional quagmire.

For years I lived to please others. Whether this was out of duty or because of my innate desire for approval, I can tell you that focusing on others really wore me down and eventually left me feeling depleted, with little drive or identity of my own. I ate uncontrollably out of poor self-esteem and lack of confidence. Though my insecurities were rooted in my childhood, they followed me right into adulthood, where life in the spotlight coupled with the extraordinary demands of royal life only exacerbated and magnified them.

Fast-forward to today and what's different? Now I live in truth, which means I trust my instincts and I follow my heart. If being untrue to myself and my needs made me weak before, I owe my strength and conviction now to the truth and authenticity I reaffirm in myself each day. I tell people

I feel as if I've become the conductor who is leading the orchestra that is my life.

I'm living proof that if you feel stuck where you are, you can reclaim your life and make it better than you'd ever imagined. First you need to pause and regroup—and this book will show you how. If you are over-weight as I was, you'll quickly see how your lifestyle, relationships and habits are affecting your sense of well-being. Don't let fear of change hold you back. From my own experience and in talking with others I have come to learn that we know *intuitively* when we're ready to face specific issues and take steps to address them. Weight Watchers practically saved me by opening my eyes to the unhealthy feelings and behaviors that were behind my eating problems *and* many of the troubles in other parts of my life. I'd never have moved on had I not already been receptive to change.

It's fair to say that I reinvented myself as a result of losing weight. I know I look better because I weigh less, but it was the weight-loss process itself that gave me the opportunity to change my life on many levels. Aside from looking different on the outside, I also have more spirit and energy on the inside. My outlook is brighter. I'm a better person and a great mother, all because my reinvention started at my very core and worked its way out-ward. I feel happier and more in control because the changes touched the very corners of my mind, body and soul. Understanding the triggers of my emotional eating was like peering into a window on myself. I used to feel victimized by the circumstances of change, but now I embrace goal setting and making the decisions that lead me toward achieving them. Now, my outlook on the future is positive because I'm the one shaping my destiny.

Reinventing Yourself is a book about learning to change—the small, as well as large, issues in your life. In these chapters we'll set out together on *your* path of rediscovery and reinvention. This is *your* time and *your* journey, so it's *your* opportunity to start focusing on how *you* feel and on what *you* want. Put all judgment aside and make today a clean slate.

The funny thing is, though, that even when you take charge and begin to experience all the rewards and reap the good feelings you experience from your efforts, something always comes up that may make you question just how far you've really come in your journey. For example, for all the positive, forward steps I've taken in the past few years, I occasionally find myself vexed by old issues, insecurities or problems. To this day, when I have a falling-out with a friend or read something hurtful about myself in the press, I still take it deeply personally and then experience the familiar spectrum of emotions—everything from anger to embarrassment to sadness. That's when I ask myself, Didn't I take care of this one already?

Working on this book and interviewing the nine Weight Watchers leaders profiled in these chapters has helped me realize something important about the process of change: We don't suddenly change ourselves and our lives. For most of us, change is an ongoing process; it doesn't just happen, and things aren't suddenly better. I often remind myself that change can be subtle—in fact, the more subtle the change, the more profound and powerful its impact. The key is not falling back into old habits; it's about reminding yourself not to opt for the familiar simply because it's what you know and what feels comfortable. With every change comes a little discomfort, but trust me: The discomfort is temporary, and soon the positive side of change will appear.

I know you'll feel inspired as you progress through this book, especially as you read the first-person success stories from the Weight Watchers leaders. I truly enjoyed interviewing each of these remarkable women. They first came to Weight Watchers as members, each with her own history but all of them feeling out of control about their weight and their lives. Things changed as these women shed pounds and reinvented healthier lives for themselves. Now they inspire hundreds each week back home where they now lead Weight Watchers meetings. What is truly wonderful about the ideas contained in this book is that you can reach whatever goals you set for yourself. Anyone can succeed with the right frame of mind. The key is to ease into the process of looking at your life and pause often to reflect on yourself. Start dreaming about your future and get excited about change, too. Good things await you.

If you're truly ready to take charge of your life or if you're tired of feeling unhappy, then dive into this book with an open mind and heart. It's most effective if you read the chapters in the order in which they appear, take the quizzes, and listen to the advice and ideas we've presented. But if you're more comfortable picking and choosing your chapters and focusing on the profiles, by all means do it that way. The key is to read, listen and learn—about your life and your true self.

I have come to think of life as a fast-flowing river. As anyone who has ever gone rafting on the rapids knows, you have to be alert to whatever you might encounter, be it storms or taking a corner too sharply and finding yourself at the brink of a terrifying waterfall. I hope this book gives you the ballast to help you the next time you feel as if you are moving too fast, losing control, and about to be thrown out of your raft.

So we're on our way now . . . down the rapids towards the mouth of the river. In these pages, I feel I've tried to show that the current can sometimes be very rough and strong, that there are days when I need to really focus to understand how best to negotiate the corners of the river up ahead. I worry so much about the storms, the waterfalls, the rough waters, but I am determined to get to my goal. Thank you for joining me in this trip together on such a wonderful river. You know how the weather can change, so let's just take one day at a time.

CHAPTER ONE

Say Hello to the Real You

ho do you think you are?" For much of my life I probably would have pulled a blank to that question. When you are a natural-born people pleaser like me, it's easy to lose touch with yourself as you focus on satisfying everyone else. Looking back, I have to wonder why I was so inattentive to my own need for happiness.

In my case, the reason is partly cultural. I was brought up in the best British tradition, where girls are raised to be modest, independent and selfless. Some of us British keep a "stiff upper lip" even in the worst of times, but I've learned that ignoring weakness is not always such a good trait. That's why I encourage my girls to recognize and feel their emotions and I teach them to deal constructively with the source of their sadness, anger or frustration.

Why is it that so many women, regardless of age and nationality, struggle so hard to hold everything together, only to lose themselves in the process? In this chapter you'll meet Weight Watchers leader Sharon Walls, whose esteem and sense of control was eroded by loneliness and the stress of raising a young family while her husband worked half a world away.

When Sharon made a conscious decision to get control of her weight she turned to Weight Watchers for help. She expected to lose weight by dieting, but the experience proved much more than that as Sharon rediscovered her needs and goals while also understanding the emotional root of her eating. We see from her story that food alone is not to blame for weight gain and that dealing with a weight problem means dealing with behavior and lifestyle issues as well.

I tell my friends that when it comes to dieting, "start with your mind and your bottom will follow." How we think really does affect who we are, which is why I'm a fan of Weight Watchers "Tools for Living," a set of wonderful techniques that help you get what you want. Sharon uses a visualization technique that lets her focus on the good feelings that she'll enjoy upon reaching a goal. This is the tool called Motivating Strategy. We've both embraced the tool we call Positive Self-Talking to better manage our "inner critic" and turn up the volume on thoughts that encourage us to succeed and feel good about ourselves.

The potential for change is in each and every one of us. Change calls for taking lessons from our past to create our future. New and better things are possible because of change, so don't let fear hold you back.

Profile: SHARON WALLS
Rethinking Who I Want to Be

For most of her adult life, Sharon Walls had been about 20 pounds overweight. She wasn't happy with the extra pounds but she could live with them. After she gave birth to her first child, and added another 25 pounds to her 5-foot 11-inch frame, she decided to do something about it. Sharon joined Weight Watchers in 1990 and lost 45 pounds without a problem. Life was good until Walls gave birth to her third child, and found herself 45 pounds overweight—again. "I felt a little smug because I'd done this before," recalls Sharon, now 42, a Weight Watchers leader in southern California. "And I thought I should be able to lose the weight all by myself. But I couldn't."

Compounding matters, the family had recently moved to southern California, the land of the slim and beautiful—and Sharon felt completely out of her element. The family had spent four years in New Zealand, where Walls had built up a wonderful support network and loved the adventure of living in a new country. "When we moved to southern California, I literally felt like I was starting from scratch again," she explains. "And there were moments when I felt like I wasn't anywhere I wanted to be. I felt invisible—I was always doing everything for everybody but I was feeling so empty inside. I was being a victim; I let everything happen to me. I was living with a just-get-through-the-day mentality, and I was totally in a stuck mode. I would dwell on negative things, such as conflicts, instead of dealing with them and moving on. But I also had a sense that there was more to life than this. I started searching for something. I was really trying to redefine who I wanted to be."

In 1996, Sharon decided to take the first step—by addressing her weight issues. "I was really at rock bottom," she recalls. "I weighed 200 pounds. My husband is a runner and very fit, and I was embarrassed to be seen with him. I had the lowest self-esteem of my life. I felt dowdy and completely out of control of my life. And I just had this feeling that if I didn't start, I would be 200 pounds for the rest of my life and I didn't want to be there." She rejoined Weight Watchers, and within nine months she'd peeled off those extra 45 pounds by changing her eating habits, exercising portion control, taking up walking, and finding other outlets (instead of turning to food) to relieve emotional frustration. "It's not just a matter of knowing what to do," she says. "It's whether you're ready to do it. And I was ready to embrace this."

Not only did Sharon lose the weight and become a Weight Watchers leader in 1997, but she was so committed to revamping her lifestyle that she joined a running club. As Walls increased her mileage and trained closely with a buddy, she set her sights on running the Los Angeles marathon in March of 1998. "It was something I really wanted to accomplish by the age of 40," she explains. "With this marathon and losing weight, it was about moving forward, instead of moving backward; about dwelling on what I was going to be instead of on what I wasn't. Before this, I was always putting my three children or my husband first and I wasn't taking care of me. I decided to become a person who took her needs into consideration. This taking care of myself helps me take care of my kids and my husband and everything else. It's a real choice. The conflicts, the demands, and the emotional upheaval are still there, but taking care of myself helps me stay centered so I can deal with it all."

Sharon got serious about training for the marathon and treated her running time as sacred. She learned to carve out time for her workouts and protected it fiercely, setting limits with other people and saying, "No, this is Sharon's hour" when necessary. "The marathon—running 26 miles after having three children—was pivotal," she recalls. "I was building an emotional bank account while I was doing my training. The stronger I felt about taking care of me, the more competent I felt about going out there and taking chances." Even with all the preparation and her positive mind-set, however, the marathon itself proved to be a formidable challenge. At the twenty-first-mile mark, Sharon's energy reserves were completely drained. "I sat down at the side of the road and cried and decided to quit," she confesses. While tears were streaming down her face, she looked up and saw a man with two prosthetic legs walking the marathon. "When I saw that, I just screamed at myself: You can do this—now get up!" she says. "I figured if he could do this without any legs, I could do this with two even if they hurt." Sure enough, Sharon got back on her feet, made herself get moving and finished the marathon.

But Sharon didn't rest on her laurels. Shortly after the marathon she enrolled in a class called Introduction to Counseling. She found it so stimulating that she decided to go back to school to earn a master's degree in marriage and family therapy. Her goal: to become a therapist. "I kept searching for what I wanted and I kept putting myself out there," she says. "It was like I kept drawing new things toward me. Going back to school has been a huge commitment and I have a lot of guilt because my kids are still young (they're three, eight and nine), but I just try to muscle through it. This is about who I am inside."

For Sharon, making one change sparked a desire to take another risk or try another experience and so on, until Sharon was well on her way to becoming who she wants to be. "Ever since I was a kid, I've been a striver," she explains. "I've always had a sense of wanting to accomplish something and give something of myself back to the world. It's a competitive spirit inside—to be the best I can be. I feel like I'm a totally different person than I was five years ago. Back then, I was looking to the outside world for my happiness and for feeling okay about myself. I look inward now for that voice that tells me what I need and what I need to do to get to a place where I feel okay. That voice helps me stay in the moment more and be more accepting of where I am, which I think is the most valuable gift I can give myself."

WHO ARE YOU? It's a simple enough question but it's often hard to answer. If you're like many women, you might say, "I'm a mother, a wife, a lawyer (or architect or accountant or whatever the case may be), a daughter, a friend, a short-order cook, a housekeeper, a laundry expert, a gardener." And while all of those answers might be true, they all reflects who you are in the eyes of other people, in terms of what you do for them or with

Your Roles, Your Well-Being

Several studies have found an association between the number of roles people occupy in their lives and their psychological well-being. One body of research has found a consistent connection between having numerous social ties and good health and psychological well-being. Another body of research suggests that juggling work and family roles promotes mental well-being. And numerous studies have found that married people tend to live longer and more healthfully than single people do.

Nevertheless, other research has found that women often respond differently to these factors than men do. For example, being employed boosts a woman's sense of well-being directly or may serve as a buffer against stress experienced in other roles (such as that of wife and mother). But it also appears that women may be especially vulnerable to role conflicts (clashes that occur when fulfilling the demands of one role jeopardizes a person's performance in another) and role overload (having so many demands related to a person's roles that performing well becomes virtually impossible).

In fact, a recent study involving 296 women who simultaneously cared for aging parents and occupied the roles of mother, wife and employee found that when women attached a greater sense of personal importance to these roles, they tended to have better psychological well-being. The theory is that people gain more meaning, a greater sense of purpose, and stronger guidance in how to behave in their lives when they're carrying out a role that they perceive to be essential to their concept of who they are. It also may be that they're more attuned to the rewards of that role. But at the same time, this sense of role importance can increase the potential for distress when the pressure mounts. Specifically, when women valued the roles of

continued on next page

wife and employee highly, they were more vulnerable to the effects of stress in these areas. (Interestingly, this wasn't true of the mother role!)

Trying to be Superwoman can be a losing proposition. Which means that it's up to you to take steps to broaden your self-definition and safeguard your emotional health. It's not just a matter of functioning well in each area of your life or warding off effects of stress. It's a matter of empowering yourself to lead a more gratifying life.

them. The truth is, you are more than the sum of your roles, responsibilities and accomplishments. None of these responses reflects who you are as a unique, separate person, and none of them addresses what makes you tick, what gets your energy flowing or what you feel passionate about in life. In short, lost in these descriptions is the sense of who you are in your own eyes, which is where it counts the most.

And that's too bad, because if you lose sight of who you are, deep down in your heart and soul, how can you possibly have a pulse on what you really want out of life? How can you feel grounded in this world? How can you make sense of your experiences? And how can you make decisions for your future?

Your image of yourself (in psychological terms it's called your self-concept) has a powerful influence on how you view the world and your life. In a nutshell, your self-concept reflects how you see yourself and what you believe about yourself. Over time, this contributes to your sense of identity. Your self-concept isn't a fixed entity, though; it can shift slightly from one situation to another, from one day to the next, depending partly on how you feel physically and emotionally. For example, you might feel full of confidence at your own birthday party, where you may be surrounded by people who know and love you. But you could feel like a mass of insecurities, possibly even downright inferior, a few days later when you're asked to brief your colleagues on a subject you know little about. In the first setting, your self-concept may be primarily positive; in the second, it could veer more toward the negative.

Self-Concept, Deconstructed

Your self-concept isn't completely dependent on the environment. On the contrary, it's a complex phenomenon that incorporates a variety of factors. Your self-concept includes personality traits—such as shyness or intelligence—that may have been present since birth. But your beliefs about yourself also develop in response to experiences and your understanding of the roles you play in your life. Moreover, your self-concept also encompasses your body image, your sense of your own worth as a human being (your self-esteem, in other words), your sense of how other people see you, your sense that with some effort you can control events in your life, and the level of acceptance you have of yourself. In addition, your values, goals, plans, attitudes and moods also affect your sense of self.

When it comes to a person's definition of herself, all of these elements are intricately intertwined. But research from Vanderbilt University has found that men and women tend to think of themselves primarily in terms of the roles they hold; indeed, the social roles they occupy are powerful sources of their self-concepts. And for many people, self-esteem also plays a starring role. In a series of studies, psychologist Jennifer D. Campbell, Ph.D., of the University of British Columbia, found that a person's self-esteem deeply influences the clarity of her self-concept; in other words, how she feels about or evaluates herself colors what she believes about herself. What Campbell discovered is that the self-concept of people with low self-esteem is more dependent on outside influences: what other people think of them or how they handle a particular situation. People with high self-esteem, in contrast, tend to have clearer, more stable self-concepts from one situation to another.

The moral of the story: If you don't have a clear sense of who or how you are, it may be worth taking steps to bolster your self-esteem. How? By accentuating the positive—particularly, your strengths and unique qualities—rather than dwelling on your weaknesses. By increasing your comfort zone by taking on challenges that are slightly out of reach but reasonable. By reminding yourself of your successes. And by facing your fears and working through them. In the process of boosting your self-esteem, you'll also be taking steps to strengthen your self-concept.

And that's worthwhile because your self-concept helps you interpret external information that's relevant to you. It helps you frame goals to guide your behavior in the future. It helps to convey a consistent image of who you are to other people. And a clear self-concept may even protect your health: A study from the University of Washington found that people with uncertain self-concepts were more vulnerable to stress-related lapses in health than were those with a strong sense of identity.

The Hazards of an Unexamined Life

If you don't have a clear sense of who you are, it may be because you've been batted around by stress and turmoil in your life or because you've grown too accustomed to looking outward, not inward. Especially in these high-speed times, it's all too easy to get swept up in the current of life and to lose sight of yourself as a separate, distinct person. It's a common hazard of leading a busy, hectic life, especially for working mothers. And it's hardly surprising when you consider that after fulfilling work responsibilities, caring for children, and completing chores at home, employed mothers have only an hour a day of personal time during the week, according to a recent survey by the Families and Work Institute in New York City. What's more, in a survey of 3,000 executives, 55 percent reported that they work at least 60 hours a week, and 29 percent confessed to 70 hours or more. No wonder 58 percent of working mothers in another survey reported that overtime work was a frequent cause of family squabbles.

When you feel pulled in multiple—and often conflicting—directions, or you're catering to the demands of too many people, it's easy to overlook your own wants and needs. Thinking about those can seem selfish or like an unaffordable luxury. Besides, when your plate is full of stress and responsibilities, sometimes it's just easier to avoid examining some of the unpleasant realities of your life—whether it's dissatisfaction with your career, your weight, your marriage or something else entirely—and simply carry on with business as usual. Indeed, many people make their way through life surrounded by a bubble of denial and self-deception. It's less painful that way. On some level, they probably figure that if they don't face the truth about a certain aspect of their lives, it won't exist. Or maybe they're secretly hoping the circumstances will magically change one day and they'll suddenly be happy. That's not likely to happen.

In all likelihood, the status quo will be maintained, and it can slowly, insidiously eat away at your sense of happiness and well-being. More often than not, continuously operating on automatic pilot eventually takes its toll, leaving you depleted of physical, emotional and spiritual energy. You could begin to suffer from depression, anxiety, stress overload, fatigue or other health conditions. Or you could wake up one day with a profound feeling of emptiness inside. None of these possibilities is good.

If there's one thing you can count on, it's this: If you don't take charge of your life, no one else will do it the way you would want him or her to. You're the director of your own show; in other words, you're accountable and responsible for your life. Of course, being passive is a choice, too, but it's one that will not serve you well in the end. After all, if you find yourself squelching your desires and simply following someone else's lead, you could wind up resenting it—and them.

Priority #1: You

The odds are, you probably already have some inkling of what you want for yourself and your life. What many people need most is permission to make themselves a priority and pursue what's really important to them. We're all works in progress. Month after month, and year after year, we're all trying—on some level, conscious or not—to figure out who we are and how we can strive to create the lives we want to live. Even so, there comes a time in many people's lives when they're ready to make significant changes, whether it's in their lifestyles, their careers or marital status, their geographical location or some other area of their lives. They might wake up one morning wondering how they arrived at the life they have. Or they may be walking around haunted by a vague sense of uneasiness. Or they may have a sudden epiphany about what they really want.

However the desire for change is sparked, the trouble is, many people don't know where or how to start to make a difference in their lives. They become so intent on moving forward that they may not be fully aware of their present circumstances or of what they really want deep down. Then they feel frustrated and disappointed when they end up with a result they hadn't quite planned on, or they don't understand why they wound up where they did.

The truth is, if you want to effectively change some aspect of your life, you have to understand what you want and why you want it. You need to chart your course toward a goal and to start altering your behavior. But before you try to change your behavior, it helps to understand why you've been doing whatever it is that you've been doing: to understand yourself, your thought patterns and habits, what motivates you, what holds you back, and so on. Without gaining this self-understanding, you'll just end up repeating the same old ways of thinking and doing and you'll feel stuck in a rut.

The journey to positive change or self-improvement has to begin in your head. Why? Because, as psychologists point out, beliefs reside in your mind, and your thoughts, ideas and attitudes, all of which originate in your mind, spur you into action and affect your perception of everything that happens. They guide your behavior. They act as a filter through which you experience situations and events. And they act as an expert commentator when it's time to analyze what has already happened. In this way, the landscape of the mind has the power to shape your entire life. For example, if you believe you can't do something—whether your goal is to lose weight, learn a new computer program or master a new sport—you probably won't be able to do it. And that's because your mind will be holding you back, discouraging you when you most need encouragement, setting up obstacles where there aren't any, or letting you give up when you need to persevere. On the other hand, if you believe your goal can be accomplished, your mind—and hence your behavior—will do nearly everything it can to help you succeed.

While research has found that women who have both a family and a career generally find their multiple roles fulfilling, conflicts inevitably arise that can cause a woman's stress level to soar. It's not a matter of perception; it's a fact. And although you can't make these conflicts go away, you can often change the way you think about them and deal with them, which can have a powerful effect in easing your burden. In a study involving married professional women with children, researchers at the University of Texas at Austin discovered that striving to meet existing role demands—by becoming more efficient and planning their time more carefully—and changing their attitudes about these work-family clashes were the most powerful coping mechanisms for handling them. Which suggests that your state of mind can be a potent ally in many aspects of your life.

If there's one thing that's entirely within your power to change, it's your attitude. As the English poet William Blake wrote in *The Marriage of Heaven and Hell,* "If the doors of perception were cleansed everything would appear to man as it is, infinite." The key, then, is to open the doors of your mind to the possibilities of life and particularly to the possibilities of change. In order to do this, you must be willing to examine life from more than one angle, to shift your point of view. But first you'll need to cultivate a sense of self-awareness, an understanding of how you see yourself now and how you view the world, then you can address how you want to develop as a person.

Putting Yourself on the List

The truth is, most women take better care of other people—their spouses, children, friends and parents—than they do themselves. It shouldn't be that way. You are just as worthy of such tender, loving care as anyone else is. Besides, why should you be continuously self-sacrificing when, chances are, no one else in your household is? As Harvard psychologist Alice Domar, Ph.D., points out in her book *Self-Nurture: Learning to Care for Yourself as Effectively as You Care for Everyone Else* (Viking/Penguin), "What women need is to learn how to nurture themselves. We need to shower as much loving kindness on ourselves as we habitually shower on loved ones . . . the only way we can have fully formed selves is by granting ourselves the same tenderness and fierce protectiveness we'd otherwise reserve for a beloved child."

Indeed, the potential benefits of self-care are enormous. Taking psychological and emotional care of yourself helps shore up your self-esteem when it might be flagging. It makes life seem more multidimensional, more manageable, and more enjoyable. It can help improve the quality of your relationships by making you less needy or stressed out. And it helps replenish energy that's been spent on everyday activities, energy you'll need to maintain motivation to make the changes in your life that you crave.

But all too often, women treat themselves as second-class citizens: We've been socialized to be sensitive to other people's needs, but many women take this to an extreme, believing, on some level, that everyone *else's* needs come before their own. And they figure that after everyone else has been taken care of, they'll finally be able to focus what's left of their time, energy and attention on their own concerns. The trouble is, there's not much left after everyone else's wants and needs have been catered to. As a result, many women end up giving themselves short shrift.

But the reality is, if you want to improve your life, you need to start with the way you take care of yourself. And the key is to make changes from the inside out. It's all well and good to try to lose weight to feel better about yourself. Or to find a more fulfilling career to give you more satisfaction in life. Or to pursue a promising relationship that provides you with a deep sense of connection. But often *real* transformation starts from within when you explore the yearnings that underlie those goals. Indeed, if you focus on taking good care of yourself, on figuring out what gives your life meaning and what your personal values are, and then find a way to get more of those good things into your life, you'll naturally gain a healthy dose of self-awareness and a clear sense of your priorities. And often feeling grounded and good about yourself can set off a cascade of subtle events that bring improvements to your life.

The Benefits of Self-Care

Let's say you embark on a regimen to eat more nutritious food and exercise regularly in an effort to improve your health: With commitment and perseverance, you may end up losing weight and feeling better about your body. This could lead to a boost in self-confidence, which could affect how you present yourself to other people and what risks—emotional and physical—you're willing to take. Because you feel stronger and more capable, you might decide to go after a job promotion or try a new sport. These pursuits might encourage you to begin networking professionally or meeting new people socially. And things might just start to happen for you in many areas of your life. At that point, it may seem magical, as though you're attracting luck. But it has less to do with simple good fortune than with taking charge of one aspect of your life and putting yourself out there. With daring to present yourself in a new way.

The good news is, self-presentation seems to take a step in a stronger, more distinctive direction as we get older. Research from Wayne State University in Detroit has found that with the passing years, adults tend to shift away from emphasizing what they have in common with others and how they conform to social conventions; instead, they increasingly present themselves as unique individuals who have a complex personal history, both psychologically and chronologically. But you don't have to wait for the hands of time to move; you can nudge your self-presentation in a more distinctive direction now.

And it's worth the effort, because when you begin to feel special and distinctive, you tend to put your best foot forward and send a confident message about yourself into the world. This can have an effect that's almost like a magnet pulling good things toward you. Have you ever noticed how "lucky" people often seem to be in the right place at the right time? How good fortune seems to smile upon them? It's not that they have any mystical secrets to their success. Indeed, psychologists have found that people who see themselves as lucky or unlucky often dwell on the aspects of their lives that support their perception, a phenomenon called selective recall. When asked to recall key moments in their history, "lucky" people reflect

How Body-Esteem Fits into Self-Esteem

Intimately connected with how you see and feel about yourself is your body image—how you see and feel about your physical self. Research from Old Dominion University in Norfolk, Virginia, has found that body image makes up about 25 percent of a person's self-esteem. A woman's perception of her own body has a more significant impact on her feelings about herself and her sense of self-worth than it does for a man; most men aren't as emotionally invested in their physical selves. If a woman is happy with her body, her movements and expressions are likely to be confident, flowing and graceful; if she feels distressed about her appearance, on the other hand, her movements and expressions may be awkward, self-conscious and constricted.

Unfortunately, the vast majority of American women are unhappy with their bodies, regardless of where they fall on the weight charts. In large measure this is due to the pressure women feel to conform to cultural standards of beauty that are depicted on television, in movies and in magazines—standards that are completely unattainable for most women. To some extent, these treat women as sexual objects, a phenomenon that can be highly damaging. In a recent study at Duke University, researchers examined the link between being preoccupied with one's own physical appearance, body shame and eating disorders. What they found is that women who were extremely focused on their physical appearance were at increased risk for disordered eating habits. The reason: They felt ashamed of their bodies. As the researchers noted, this body shame can, in turn, have a profoundly negative impact on a woman's sense of self.

But not every woman who feels dissatisfied with her body suffers from disordered eating habits or a poor sense of self. Indeed, recent

continued on next page

research from the University of Wisconsin–Madison has found that women who harbor a negative view of their bodies but have normal eating habits tend to have healthier coping strategies—problem solving, seeking social support, reducing tension, emphasizing the positive—which help them cope with not feeling as well as they could about themselves physically. They're also better able to isolate their poor body image so that it doesn't affect their broader view of themselves. In other words, they're able to maintain positive beliefs about themselves, even if they don't always feel comfortable in their own skin.

Once again, these results highlight just how important it is to have an expansive view of yourself, one that allows you to feel positively about many different facets of yourself and your life.

on the situations that made them feel fortunate, and this focus perpetuates their ability to see themselves in a positive way.

In other words, luck has less to do with whether you're smiled upon by Fortune than with how you view your experiences. It also has to do with your approach to life—how much control you feel you have, how independent and persistent you are, whether you know when to cut your losses, and, of course, how you present yourself to the world. Lucky people capitalize on opportunities that appear for them and they do the necessary legwork to prepare for challenges. Among the key elements in luck's existence is a trait called self-efficacy—a can-do spirit and a sense of self-confidence that give you the gumption to strive for what you want. People with a strong sense of self-efficacy feel in control of their fate. They figure out what they want, set goals, work hard at achieving them, and notice promising opportunities. They're not afraid to go after what they want because they've made themselves a priority in their lives. They treat themselves as if they were special and often present themselves as lucky to other people. In other words, they create their own luck, and it has a transforming effect on them in the process.

Assessing Yourself

Before you can take steps toward enhancing your sense of yourself or improving your life, you need to get reacquainted with your strengths, your weaknesses, your hopes, your dreams. Think of it as a way of becoming intimately familiar with your inner world. This self-awareness will serve as a prelude to change. Chances are, your inner landscape has changed from what it was, say, 5, 10 or 20 years ago. So it's time to update the picture with a little self-exploration. Get out a pen and pad of paper or a journal book, and do the following exercises.

Self-Exploration Exercise #1: My Life in Review

Choose a time when you're not rushed, when you have the luxury of being alone with your own thoughts, and ask yourself these 20 questions. Write down the answers; they hold valuable lessons: They can help you frame your actions, set priorities and overcome stumbling blocks as you pursue new goals.

1. Am I doing what I want to do with my career—or am I doing what's easy or comfortable?

2. What would I consider my ideal job or vocation?

3. What's my greatest triumph in life so far?

Coming to Terms with Disappointment

As you review your life and your dreams, you may feel a sense of disappointment. Even if you've achieved many of the things you thought you wanted—buying a house, getting a new job, marrying and starting a family—you may feel unfulfilled. And if you feel chronically disappointed—over the loss of your dreams or the failure of your expectations, for example—this can affect your general attitude toward life and lead to feelings of sadness, anger, or despair, according to psychologist David Brandt, Ph.D., author of *Is That All There Is? Balancing Expectation and Disappointment in Your Life* (Impact).

But there are valuable lessons in disappointment, which is basically nothing more than unmet expectations or the loss of an anticipated outcome. If you examine your disappointments and your pattern of becoming disappointed and express your feelings about them (individually or collectively), you can often uncover your true desires in life. The key is to first reveal your underlying expectation and then to ask yourself why it's important to you. For example, if you recently felt disappointed by the squabbling that went on at a family reunion and you examine how and why you feel let down, you might realize that what you really want is to have a family that gets along; on a deeper level, you might discover that what you truly crave is a sense of peace in your life. Then, if you examine this desire objectively, you might realize how unrealistic it is to expect an extended family to get along famously all the time. Once you accept that, you can let go of your dashed hopes and the downward emotional pull they can exert.

After you've moved away from the feeling, you might also start to think about ways to modify your expectations so that they are

continued on next page

more realistic in the future. Or you might consider how you can take steps to attain your underlying desire on your own. If a sense of peace is what you crave, for instance, you might pursue avenues that lead to developing inner peace—learning to meditate or do yoga, taking nature walks or keeping a journal—instead of expecting a sense of calm to prevail in the external world. The bottom line is: If handled the right way, disappointment can actually inspire you to take steps toward improving your life.

4. What is my most precious unrealized dream?

5. Do I have a secret ambition?

6. Who in my life has had the most profound influence on me?

7. How do I want to live?

8. What's been the biggest disappointment or trauma in my life so far and how has it shaped me?

9. What do I fear most in life?

10. What would I do if my worst fear actually happened?

11. What makes me feel most competent in my life?

12. What special ingredient seems to be missing from my life?

13. Where do I pour most of my time and energy?

14. If I didn't have to work, how would I choose to spend my time?

15. What activity makes me feel happiest and most fulfilled?

16. How would I describe the ideal marriage?

17. How would I most like people to remember me after I'm gone?

_____

_____

18. What would I most like to change about myself?

_____

_____

19. How would I describe my philosophy of life? Am I following it?

_____

_____

20. If I could rewrite one part of my history, what would it be?

_____

_____

Self-Exploration Exercise #2: Where Your Energy Goes Versus Where You Want It to Go

To figure out how you currently divide your time and energy into different aspects of your life, draw a pie chart like the one below. Draw lines wherever you see fit to indicate how much of your life—and yourself—is devoted to your career, your marriage (or romance, if you're single), your children, your parents, your friends, home management, physical activity, other leisure activities, self-care, volunteer or civic duties, spirituality, and other pursuits.

Next, draw another circle and divide it to indicate how much of yourself, your time and energy, you'd like to spend in the 8 to 10 aspects of your life that you value most. These can include your career, romance, family, friends, hobbies, fitness or other health activities, spiritual pursuits, community involvement, or something else altogether (but be specific about what it is).

Now, compare your two circles. Note the discrepancies in how you spend your precious time and energy. For each area where there's a con-

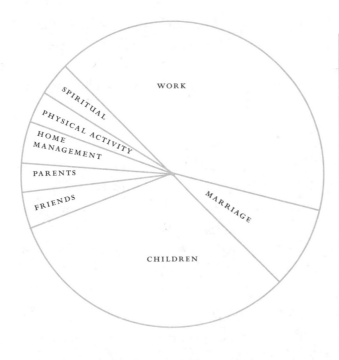

THE ELEMENTS
Work
Marriage
Children
Parents
Friends
Home
management
Physical
activity
Other leisure
activities
Self-Care
Volunteer or
civic duties
Spiritual
renewal
Other

siderable difference, write down two things that you can start doing now to improve that area of your life. In the area of romance, this might include making a weekly lunch date with your honey or spending 20 minutes catching up on each other's lives after the kids go to bed. In the area of spiritual pursuits, this could include spending 15 minutes a day in solitude, thinking about your values and beliefs or meditating, or taking a class in religious studies. In the area of fitness, you might choose to take a walk twice a week during your lunch hour or sign up for a spinning or yoga class one night a week. By mapping out things you can do to improve various aspects of your life now, you'll see that you do have the power to make small but effective changes that will add up to significant improvements over time.

Self-Exploration Exercise #3: Facing the Mirror

If you were to look at yourself as a friend might look at you, who would you see? Read through all the qualities that are listed below and next to each indicate how well they describe you as you are today. Rate them on a scale from 1 to 3—with 1 indicating "very descriptive of me," 2 meaning "somewhat descriptive of me," and 3 being "not at all descriptive of me." This will help you create an honest but uncritical profile of what you believe about yourself today.

Note: Save your answers because you will refer to this self-evaluation again later.

Caring	*Patient*	*Friendly*	*Gentle*
Energetic	*Creative*	*Articulate*	*Cooperative*
Clever	*Resilient*	*Likable*	*Independent*
Resourceful	*Intelligent*	*Assertive*	*Spontaneous*
Passionate	*Considerate*	*Lighthearted*	*Ambitious*
Funny	*Reliable*	*Organized*	*Thoughtful*
Playful	*Tactful*	*Warm*	*Competent*

Self-Exploration Exercise #4: Rating Your Perceptions of Yourself

Now that you have a clearer sense of how you see yourself, it's time to evaluate what you see. Based on your perceptions of yourself, take a look at your traits and honestly assess those you like and those you don't by answering the following questions:

1. Write down the three qualities you most like about yourself.

2. Why do you like each of them?

3. How do you use these qualities in your life?

4. How could you put them to further use in your life, to improve yourself or gain new opportunities for personal growth?

_____

_____

5. Write down the three qualities you least like about yourself.

_____

_____

_____

6. Why don't you like each of them?

_____

_____

7. How has each of these qualities influenced your life, for better or worse?

_____

_____

8. What, if anything, could you do to change or improve them?

_____

_____

_____

Hopefully, you've gained some insights into yourself with this exercise. But it's also important to put these insights into practice by taking steps to use your positive qualities more effectively or to improve upon the less desirable ones. Make a conscious effort to take small steps in these directions daily.

Self-Exploration Exercise #5: How Do You Operate?

Now you've got a pulse on your values and your personality traits. But a key question is: How are you putting these insights to use? Use this questionnaire to assess how you generally conduct yourself in your life. For this exercise, ask two close friends or loved ones to answer these questions about you, too.

- Do you generally act in accordance with a strong sense of purpose or a philosophy of life?

- How well do you prepare mentally and emotionally for challenges that lie ahead?

- Are you effective at managing your time—or does it manage you?

- How well do you deal with adversity or unforeseen crises?

- Is your attitude generally positive and constructive, or negative and critical?

- How well do you bounce back from disappointment or setbacks?

- Do you take time for yourself—for mental or emotional refreshment—each day?

- How do you manage stress?

- Does your life have a healthy balance between work and pleasure, between social involvement and introspection?

- Generally speaking, do you feel that you have the power to control your life or do you see yourself more as a victim of circumstances, constantly reacting to whatever life throws your way?

After answering all these questions, go back through this list and look at your patterns. Use your friends' evaluations as a reality check: If there's a discrepancy between your response and theirs, take a closer look at your own behavior. If you feel comfortable doing so, it may even be helpful to discuss their perceptions of your behavior with them. They may see you doing things that you're not aware of.

Next, jot down at least two things you could do to improve upon what you've been doing in each area. For example, if you don't usually prepare well for challenges that lie ahead, think of what you could start doing— whether it's developing contingency plans in case something goes wrong, or mentally rehearsing how you might deal with potential obstacles. Similarly, if your attitude tends to gravitate toward the negative, critical end of the spectrum, think about how you could steer it back toward the middle or positive end—by making an effort to look for the silver lining in distressing situations or by using more encouraging thoughts to refute negative ones, for instance. If you practice taking these steps on a regular basis, soon enough they'll become second nature. And you'll be on your way to achieving a better you.

Putting Yourself on the Agenda

Why spend time doing all these exercises? Because they'll help you begin to see yourself in a clearer light. They'll help you rediscover what makes you tick, what gets your creative or intellectual juices flowing, what once-treasured aspects of yourself you may have lost touch with. Hopefully, these exercises will also give you a clearer picture of your values and of what's truly important to you in your life. You might just realize that it isn't what you thought it was.

When you take a step back from your day-to-day existence and reflect on all these different aspects of yourself and your life, you'll begin to see that you're greater than the sum of your parts. That there's more to you than being a wife, a mother, a working woman; that there are valuable traits and cherished dreams inside you that deserve to be nurtured. And that you deserve to carve out time and devote resources to allowing yourself to become the best you that you can possibly be.

After all, this is your life—and it's the only one you're going to get. So why not give yourself permission to make taking care of yourself and pursuing your dreams a top priority? Remind yourself that it sure beats the alternative—feeling exhausted or unhappy, or flirting with burnout, in which case you won't be much use to yourself or to those who depend on you. But if you do make self-care a priority—and learn to set limits with other people in order to do so—you'll be setting up a win-win proposition for everybody. Chances are, you'll feel happier, stronger, and more grounded in the world; you might even gain a sense of peace within yourself. And as a result, you'll probably have more energy, patience, attention, tolerance and goodwill to give your loved ones and friends. What could be better than that?

ASSIGNMENT Write a blatantly honest obituary for yourself as you are today. Put in as much detail as possible about your accomplishments, your strengths and weaknesses, your values, the qualities that make you unique, how you've lived your life, and how friends and loved ones are likely to remember you. Then take some time to reflect on how you feel about the person you've just described. Do you like her? What would you want to change about her if you could?

CHAPTER TWO

Dare to Dream a Little

Imagine how dark life would be without dreams! To me, dreams are the pixie dust that lets us think big thoughts and reach for the stars. There's something funny about dreams, though: While they are vivid and plentiful when we're happy, they become colorless if not elusive when we're not. There have been times in my life when I didn't dare to dream because my future frightened me. I've since come to see dreams as good medicine for the mind, body and spirit.

My daughters, Beatrice and Eugenie, are prolific little dreamers and I urge them to free their imaginations and watch them soar. I treasure the evenings we spend together cuddled up in bed as we take turns dreaming aloud. It's times like these that our deepest hopes seem crystal clear and everything and anything seems possible.

Have you stopped dreaming? If you have, I know Weight Watchers leader Jean Krueger's story will change that. Jean's story is a testament to the power of the human spirit in the face of real adversity. Jean was living a nightmare and it's easy to see why it was depression, not dreamy slumber, that made it so hard for her to get out of bed each day. Her wake-up call to change was a photograph so humiliating that it shook Jean out of her complacency and into action—a decision that literally turned around her health and her life.

Some dreams are pure fantasy, while others are almost like a roadmap. Jean joined Weight Watchers and was already shedding pounds when she tried some light exercise to help her progress. As the pounds came off something amazing happened. Jean no longer felt tired and overwhelmed all the time, and she even took pleasure in walking along the beach and riding her bike each day. Before long Jean was setting and achieving goals for longer and longer bike rides, eventually working her way up to a popular 50-mile stretch of road near her home in southern California. What's more amazing is that many of Jean's medical problems all but vanished, leaving her feeling 20 years younger.

At all my visits to Weight Watchers meetings, I have always stressed how vital fitness is as part of an overall weight-loss strategy. I surely would not have achieved or maintained my weight-loss goals without making fitness a priority in my life. Listening to Jean made me realize the human body is drawn to exercise, and the good feeling that comes with being conditioned to fitness helps us stick with our regimen. I've come to enjoy the time I devote to fitness, which I find brings a meditative state similar to dreaming. That's when all the day's worries seem to fall into perspective for me and I can suddenly work them out, all while I am toning up my body.

Dreams can take you on fantastic rides through the country or deep into the sea, as Jean also discovered when she took up scuba diving. When you see new possibilities your whole outlook on life changes. Losing weight won't solve all your problems, but I've found that a healthy lifestyle is enough for me to face most challenges and dream of what's yet to come.

Profile: JEAN KRUEGER
Giving Myself Permission to Soar

Though she'd struggled with her weight ever since college days filled with bratwurst, beers, and fast food, and though she'd joined Weight Watchers three different times, it wasn't until Jean Krueger saw a photograph of herself in January of 1998 that she realized just how much weight she'd really gained. "It was a big wake-up call," confesses Jean, now 56, a Weight Watchers ambassador and group leader in southern California. "I realized how heavy I'd become. I realized that I was as heavy as my mother was when she died, and she probably died from weight-related causes."

Before that defining moment, Jean had been in denial about her own struggle with the scale. When she surpassed her husband's weight, her solution was simply to stop weighing herself for an entire year. "I used to wait to get out of bed until my husband left the room," she recalls, "because I didn't want him to see me struggle to get out of bed." When her health problems mounted—first she suffered from hypertension and high cholesterol, then she was diagnosed with kidney cancer and faced an arduous recovery; and later, she was hit with arthritis and heel spurs—she did the best she could to cope but gained more weight. Then came an incredibly dark period in her life: Within a short span of time, Jean lost three brothers (two to AIDS, one to suicide), as well as her mother and father, and she entered a state of perpetual mourning. "I felt like I was continually bleeding inside," she recalls. "Food was my friend, my source of comfort. And I was trying to stuff something I could never stuff—a hole in my heart."

As Jean continued to pack on more pounds, "I just started wearing bigger muumuus and didn't want to admit I was growing in sizes," she says. "When I saw that picture of myself in January of 1998, it was the last straw. I had thought my weight gain was my little secret, but I finally realized the whole world was aware of it, too."

Once this realization set in, she joined Weight Watchers immediately, and over the course of the following year peeled 59 pounds off her 5-foot 5-inch frame. It wasn't easy—she began faithfully writing down everything she ate, reading everything she could get her hands on about nutrition and weight loss, and exercising regularly—but it was worth all the effort. "I'm convinced I got back about 20 years of my life," says Jean, who has two grown children and a granddaughter. "I knew I had to change my ways. In the past, I was unsuccessful because I guess I thought it would all happen by osmosis."

Miraculously, after slimming down, all of Jean's health problems have disappeared and she now leads an incredibly active lifestyle. While she was losing weight, her group leader suggested that Jean incorporate exercise into her life. She began by walking on the beach and riding her bike, then she set her sights on doing the Rosarita-Ensenada 50-mile fun bike ride in southern California. Achieving that goal—four times now!—felt so good that Jean began to consider other challenges she wanted to try, along with other dreams she may have been squelching when she was heavy. "I went back in my head and thought about being a kid again—what I wanted to do, things I'd always wanted to try," she recalls. The next thing she knew, she and her husband were in a pool, learning to scuba dive. "I had to get past a lot of fears but it was something I'd always dreamed about because I love fish and the sea life," Jean says. Before long, she and her husband became certified scuba divers and took a trip to the Grand Caymans. "We dove down 100 feet and saw incredible corals, fish, and stingrays," she recalls. "It was like we were in a science fiction movie and we were the stars." For her next feats, Jean wants to try kayaking and in-line skating.

In fact, losing weight has become a catalyst for all kinds of challenges Jean wants to tackle in her life. "I'm trying to change on all levels—physically, intellectually, emotionally, socially and spiritually," she explains. "I feel like I'm not done yet, and it's really kind of exciting because I don't know what's going to happen next. I'm continuing to motivate myself to strive to be the best person I can be. Intellectually, I'm trying to be open to all things. I read more than I used to, I keep abreast of the stock market, and I listen to motivational tapes all the time. I have friends in my life who are positive and supportive; I want to surround myself with positive people who help me grow. And I try to take stock of how I can be a better friend, a better wife and a better listener—by being me. I look at the glass as being half full or I see the best in people rather than things I might have been judging them for in the past.

"I had no idea what the benefits of getting slim were," she adds. "Waddling around with all that weight imprisoned me in so many ways. I'm active now and healthy, and my energy level is amazing. I still look twice when I see my reflection; I continually wonder, Who is that woman wearing my dress? But I've also found that I could change myself on many levels; I've found that there are more facets to me and more places I can take myself. I used to put myself on a treadmill and not really take the time to enjoy life. It was always rush, rush, rush. I'd never stopped to think about my goals and shape them. Now I do. I react to people and things so differently these days; I don't have the bad feelings I used to. And I take time to think about what I'm thankful for. I keep a gratitude journal, and each night before I go to bed, I write down five things I'm grateful for that happened that day."

Indeed, in the last four years, Jean has basically turned her dreams into reality, one that she treasures deeply. "I feel as though I've gone through a metamorphosis," she explains. "The roly-poly caterpillar is gone and in its place is a butterfly. I've got a new life, a whole new me. When I look back on it, I don't think I really liked myself when I was heavy. Now I like myself a lot, and I love my life. I think I used to use *food as a substitute for really living. Now, I feel like I'm bingeing on life, like I just can't get enough of life itself."*

WHAT DO YOU WANT to be when you grow up? Remember how often you were asked that question as a kid? Back then, it was absolutely thrilling to let your mind wander over the various possibilities of an older version of you—perhaps as a mother, an artist, a doctor, an actress, maybe even as an astronaut. It was a bit like playing dress-up in your mind, trying on different occupations and identities, gauging how they felt. Then you grew up and became whatever it is that you became and that was probably it (unless you've already changed careers or gone through a divorce or personal crisis that caused you to alter your life dramatically). People stopped asking what you wanted to be—and you may have stopped thinking about it. Somehow there's this idea that once you become an adult, you're cooked; you're a finished product, a mostly completed canvas. And there isn't much room for tinkering.

It shouldn't be that way. As the Russian-born activist Emma Goldman once noted, "When we can't dream any longer, we die." She wasn't speaking literally, of course, but metaphorically. And she was right: When you stop imagining the possibilities, your opportunities for personal growth suddenly shrivel, and that can make your life feel limited, perhaps even tightly constricted. On the other hand, when you really do look at the world with your eyes wide open and consider all your options, life seems expansive and much more exciting. It's not just a question of choosing a vocation, though. It's about what kind of a person you want to be—in mind, body and spirit. It's about how you want to live and what you're willing to do to make that dream become reality.

Envisioning the Ideal You

Contrary to warnings your parents may have given you as a child, daydreaming about or imagining yourself as the person you'd most like to become isn't an idle exercise. In fact, it's a necessary initial step in thinking about your potential and in charting your goals for the future. Indeed, some psychologists have explored the notion of what they call "possible selves": the ideal selves that individuals would very much like to become—or the feared selves they would like to avoid becoming. These images are, of course, in the eye of the beholder. One woman's ideal self might be someone who is creative, self-confident, thin, and well loved by her family and friends, whereas another woman might be more focused on becoming rich and famous and living in the public eye.

These same women might harbor images of their negative possible selves at some level in their minds as well. One woman might dread the thought of growing up and becoming just like her mother, whom she views as selfish, overweight, depressed, and lonely. Another might fear failing professionally and becoming destitute. These fears represent what these individuals are afraid of becoming or what they want to avoid becoming at any cost.

Whatever the details are, psychologists have found that these imagined possibilities can be powerful motivating forces in a number of ways. For one thing, if you harness these images in your mind's eye, they can serve as incentives to change and guides for your behavior in the future. While envisioning yourself as the person you'd like to become, for example, you can mentally rehearse various behaviors and courses of action to see how they'd feel. These imagined possibilities can be useful, whether they're positive or negative: You might use an image of yourself as a high-powered corporate executive (if that's your concept of your ideal self) to fuel your way through business school at night; on the other hand, you might conjure up an image of yourself stuffed into an excessively snug skirt (the dreaded overweight self) to dissuade yourself from having second helpings at a party.

Imagine the Possibilities

Before you read any further, take a few moments to picture the ideal you. Be as concrete and specific as you can; if you really stop to think about it, ideas will surely come to mind. Maybe you'd like to have more energy on a daily basis, or be more willing to take smart chances in your life. Maybe you'd like to be more assertive in the professional arena, or be more outgoing in social situations. Then again, maybe you'd like to put your creative talents to work as an artist or designer.

Whatever qualities you'd like to cultivate, jot them down in a wish list. (If you get stuck, it might help to revisit the list of traits in Self-Exploration Exercise #3 in Chapter 1 and pick ones you'd like to develop.) Be as specific as possible with each goal and give yourself a reason for each one. This way, you'll know what to work on—and you'll enhance your motivation because you'll have a strong personal incentive for those goals. After all, if you don't fully understand why you're reaching for a particular goal, how can you keep striving for it when life's circumstances divert you? Here's a glimpse at what a sample wish list might look like.

The ideal me would:

- Be better at saying no to projects or invitations I don't truly care about.
  Why I want this: So I can have more time to myself and feel less overcommitted in my life.

- Have a more upbeat attitude toward life in general.
  Why I want this: Because I'd feel happier and have more energy.

- Be able to stay calmer under pressure and handle crises more smoothly.
  Why I want this: Because this would help me think more clearly and perhaps make smarter decisions when the going gets tough.

- Have the courage to start my own consulting business.
  Why I want this: Because then I could truly do what I love and have the flexible schedule that I crave.

- Lose weight and become physically strong and fit.
  Why I want this: Because I'd live a longer, healthier life, maybe even long enough to celebrate my fiftieth wedding anniversary or to see my grandchildren grow up.

- Feel confident in a wider array of situations.
  Why I want this: So that I could meet new people easily and not be afraid of trying novel experiences.

- Be highly disciplined and proactive in many areas of my life.
  Why I want this: Because this would help me be a better ally to myself in striving for my goals, whether it's losing weight or finding a new job.

Forcing yourself to think about why you want to be a certain way that doesn't come naturally is an absolutely crucial step. Think of it as questioning your motives; it's a mistake to trust them unthinkingly. Why? Because unless you know that you have a strong and valid reason for pursuing that goal, your motivation is likely to fizzle when the process of change becomes discouraging. It's also possible that you could wind up disappointed in the end result of these changes if your expectations were out of line. For example, you may be shocked to discover that you could actually reach your goal—whether it's losing 15 pounds or starting your own business—and then find out that it alone won't make you happy. And if you realize this too late, after all your painstaking efforts have led you to your goal, you could start to backslide and undo some of the good work that you've already done. So if you want to lose weight, ask yourself *why* you want to slim down. If the underlying reason is to attract a mate, you may be able to achieve that goal in other ways. But if you think the only way to do that is to lose weight or earn more money, you could be setting yourself up for a serious fall if you don't suddenly meet the man of your dreams. In short, it's not enough to pinpoint exactly what your goals are; it's also essential to understand why they are important to you and whether your expectations are realistic.

Trying On a New Skin, Sloughing Off the Old

Viewed in a certain light, much of a person's development can be seen as a continual process of defining and achieving certain possible selves, and shedding or resisting others. By selecting, discarding and constructing various incarnations of our possible selves, we can all act as active, invested managers in our own development. After all, these possible selves are a reflection of our ideas, beliefs and visions about our potential; they incorporate our hopes, goals, dreams and fears. They become the very embodiment of who we want to be, and, if used correctly, they can help steer us in that direction.

In a study involving 210 men and women, researchers at the University of Michigan and the University of Washington explored how a person's imagined possibilities for him- or herself affected how these people see themselves and what they believe about themselves. The researchers used a questionnaire that asked about personal qualities (intelligence, creativity and the like); physical descriptions (good-looking, athletic, etc.); lifestyle possibilities (having an active social life, being health conscious, and so on); general abilities (being able to cook well or fix things, for example); potential occupational options (such as Supreme Court justice or business executive); and possible assessments that are directly linked to the opinions of others (being loved, feared, appreciated and so on). Overall, people were four times more likely to envision positive selves than negative ones. In fact, the researchers noted, "Virtually all respondents thought it was possible for them to be rich, admired, successful, secure, important, a good parent, in good shape, and to travel the world."

And yet, these possible selves were hardly identical to the way these people currently viewed themselves. Whereas nearly 97 percent of the people thought it was possible for them to be in good shape, only 67 percent currently considered themselves physically fit. Similarly, 80 percent of people thought it was possible that they'd become good public speakers, but only 59 percent thought they currently were. Not surprisingly, people who had positive images of themselves in the future tended to have more positive states of mind currently, as well as higher self-esteem and a stronger sense of personal control over their lives. Taken together, these results suggest that daring to dream about how you'd like to be can positively affect your current mood, and it could even promote a can-do spirit if it's used the right way. As the researchers noted, "positive possible selves can be exceedingly liberating because they foster hope that the present self is not immutable."

Indeed, keeping a vision of your ideal self in mind can enhance your performance in various areas of your life. Research has found, for example, that when people describe what they are *optimally* capable of doing in a particular situation rather than what they *usually* do, they tend to perform better when that situation actually arises. It's the mind-body connection, and it's especially powerful if you use all your senses to envision the scene. For example, if you mentally rehearse giving a speech before a group of people, and you imagine how the room looks, sounds, smells and feels to you, *and* you picture exactly how you want to deliver your talk, you can train your brain to do it that way when the time comes.

The Risks of Raising the Bar Too High

Using your vision of the self you'd like to become as a way of making meaningful changes in your life is an effective tool, but there is a danger in holding yourself too rigidly to this image. Studies at New York University have found that focusing on the discrepancies between the real you and the ideal you can lead to emotional upset: When researchers evaluated the different ways in which people view themselves (in terms of how they actually are, how they'd like to be, and how they think they should be) and how these different images vary, they discovered that a wide gap between the two images was associated with something like an emotional hangover. The wider the gap between the real and ideal selves (based on a woman's hopes, wishes or aspirations for herself in the future), the more likely a woman was to feel sad, disappointed or dejected after completing a task. A wide gap between the real and ideal selves (based on her beliefs about her duties, responsibilities or obligations) was associated with an increased likelihood that she would feel afraid, anxious or agitated.

How can you avoid this? By enjoying your life as it is now but continuing to strive to become the person you want to be. It's fine to aim high in your aspirations—but not so high that you've set your sights on unattain-

Becoming the New You

Imagine the ideal you by incorporating the aspects of yourself that you like (refer to Chapter 1 if you need to be reminded of what those are) with qualities you'd like to cultivate. Think about how that person would feel, how she'd act, how she'd walk, talk and dress. It might even help to identify a few people whose style and qualities resemble your image of the ideal you and watch how they handle themselves in various situations.

Once you have a vivid image of your ideal self, imagine how you would feel and act if you already were that way. Consciously spend a week practicing acting as if you already were the talented, put-together woman that you want to be—and do it in public. If you get stuck, take a cue from one of the people you admire and "borrow" their traits when you need them most: If you feel nervous about hosting a party, you might think about acting like an outgoing friend who throws fabulous parties. Similarly, if you feel out of your element at a job interview, try impersonating a colleague who's self-assured and assertive. Doing this will actually help you nudge your self-concept in the direction you want it to move. How? Because if you act the part, other people will begin to perceive and respond to you as if you really are that way. And ever so gradually you'll begin to feel as if you've transformed into the person you want to be.

When you picture the ideal you, try to do so in every aspect of your life—personal, professional, emotional and spiritual. It makes sense that if you expand your definition of yourself and broaden your interests, you'll reap opportunities for greater fulfillment in life. But this broadening of your horizons also has a protective effect on your emotional well-being: When you invest yourself in many different facets of your life, then when things go wrong in one area, you have other areas from which to draw sustenance, support,

continued on next page

distraction, and satisfaction. When you lead a well-rounded life, a crisis in one area—if your finances are in disarray, for example—doesn't upset the apple cart of your entire world. Chances are you'll be able to isolate the problem and rely on the other aspects of your life to sustain you during even an especially challenging period.

Of course, you don't want to overdo it. Spreading yourself too thin—by committing to too many projects at once or trying to squeeze too many activities into an already packed schedule—can wind up draining your energy or causing unnecessary stress and anxiety. And that defeats the purpose of what you're trying to do. The key is to set priorities and strive for a balanced, realistic and *livable* lifestyle.

able or unrealistic goals. In that case, you'll simply set yourself up for an emotional fall. All of this is a delicate balancing act, to be sure, but don't be too hard on yourself. As the nineteenth-century English essayist Thomas Carlyle once noted, "The ideal is in thyself, the impediment too is in thyself." So don't let self-criticism—or even self-evaluation—thwart your attempts to better yourself. After all, you're already halfway toward the ideal you because you're already you.

Ultimately, the best way to use your ideas of how you'd like to be is with flexibility. Your image of your ideal self can help you frame goals, help spur you into action, assist you in making decisions, and help you maintain motivation for making meaningful changes in your life. It can even help you sidestep situations that could lead you in the wrong direction. But remember, this image is just a guide. It's important to allow yourself room to grow in ways that your image of your ideal self may not include. Besides, your image of your ideal self is likely to change from time to time—and that's healthy. If you don't roll with these shifts, or if you stick too closely to your initial ideal, you'll wind up limiting yourself in yet another way.

The Right to Pursue Happiness

The pursuit of happiness is often viewed as a fundamental human right. But surprisingly enough, true happiness is less a result of personal circumstances than a reflection of a person's attitude and approach to life. (Studies suggest, for example, that lottery winners gain only a temporary jolt of joy.) So what exactly is real happiness? In recent decades, scientists have begun to study the roots of happiness (they generally refer to it as "subjective well-being") and they've uncovered some surprises. Real happiness can be defined as a pervasive sense that life is good, an ongoing perception that life is meaningful, fulfilling and, for the most part, pleasant.

Upon closer examination, psychologists have found that happy people have certain traits in common—namely high self-esteem, a sense of personal control, a sense of optimism and a strong social network. They tend to have challenging work lives that are balanced with active personal lives, and a faith that involves community support, a sense of purpose, and a sense of hope. Not surprisingly, happy people are usually in good moods, and they smile often. And, at least compared to unhappy people, happy folks tend to be more loving, forgiving, trusting, energetic, decisive, creative, sociable and helpful, according to research by David G. Myers, Ph.D., a professor of psychology at Hope College in Michigan, and Ed Diener, Ph.D., a professor of psychology at the University of Illinois. As Dr. Myers notes, "People who like and accept themselves feel good about life in general."

It's not that their lives are always easy. But happy people often use hardship as an opportunity to reevaluate their priorities, to gauge whether they're spending their time the way they really want to. Not only does this proactive approach help carry them through difficult times, but it often helps them improve their lives in the process. Indeed, happy people tend to believe that they determine their own destinies. They take responsibility for their lives and believe that with some effort they can control them. Yet they keep their goals and expectations reasonable: They're optimistic enough to have hope but they're also realistic enough to be able to distinguish between what they can control and what they can't. And they focus their attention and effort on what they can.

The Vital Force Within You

There's a close cousin to subjective well-being (aka happiness) that can actually have a synergistic effect on a person's overall sense of physical and emotional well-being. Psychologists call it subjective vitality and it refers to a person's conscious experience of possessing energy, enthusiasm and aliveness. Different cultures have similar notions of a vital energy or life force from which people can draw for physical, emotional, and spiritual health—it's called *Chi* in Chinese, *Ki* in Japanese, *Bayu* in Balinese. Subjective vitality, by slight contrast, refers to an intrinsic energy that a person feels to be her own.

The truth is, subjective vitality is more than just a feeling. It can be a powerful ally in helping you reach your goals and fulfill your dreams. For example, researchers from the University of Rochester and the University of Southern Utah have found that subjective vitality is associated with self-motivation and maintained weight loss among people who were being treated for obesity; they also found that participants who had stuck with an exercise program two years later reported greater subjective vitality. Other studies have found that positive feelings of energy are associated with less negative evaluations of an individual's personal problems.

Not surprisingly, subjective vitality is associated with greater emotional well-being and self-esteem. But it also appears to be linked with self-actualization (a person's experience of her development and expression of her self) and with self-determination (a feeling that your behavior is actually chosen by you, rather than imposed by an external source). These links suggest that by choosing to take steps to change your habits or your life, or to develop certain qualities in yourself, you've begun a process that can actually boost your sense of inner vitality as well as your general satisfaction with life.

Some psychologists believe that happiness is partly genetically determined, that we're all born with a set-point for happiness, but that we can influence it through our behavior and attitudes. One of the best ways to improve your self-image, along with your happiness quotient, is to play the part—and pretend that you feel confident, optimistic, outgoing, or whatever quality you'd like to cultivate: Research has found that acting as if you are a certain way can help create the actual feeling. For example, when researchers asked people to write essays or to present themselves to an interviewer in either a self-promoting or self-deprecating fashion, those who acted as if they were remarkably smart, caring, and sensitive later expressed higher self-esteem when they were interviewed by another researcher. What's more, studies have found that when people are instructed or induced to smile, their moods take a turn for the cheerier and they actually feel happier afterwards. How can this be? One theory is that as you observe your own behavior, you infer that you must be feeling that way; another theory maintains that smiling creates some sort of physiological feedback within the brain that then ignites the genuine feeling. Whatever the mechanism may be, psychologists agree: Forcing yourself to go through the motions can actually spark the real emotions. And this is true whether you want to feel happier, more confident, more assertive, or more lighthearted.

The Power of Decisions

In a sense, your life is the sum of all the choices and decisions you've made so far. Of course, you didn't chose to be born, and many of the decisions in your formative years were made for you by parents, teachers and other caretakers. But ever since you reached adulthood, you've had the power to make all the choices and decisions in your life—or you've allowed someone else to make them for you. Even being passive is a choice.

As with most things in life, there are good choices and bad choices. And they occur in every aspect of life—from the mundane (what to wear today, what to eat for breakfast) to the significant (Should I marry this man? Should I take this job offer?). Many of us aren't even aware of how many

Boosting Your Capacity for Happiness

It's no secret that making dramatic changes can be a slow, arduous process, whether you're trying to improve your personal life, cultivate a new career, lose weight or enhance your health. But there's good news: While you're striving to make significant changes to your life, you can also take small steps to increase your senses of happiness, fulfillment and inner vitality. This emotional upswing will, in turn, make the process of change less stressful. Here are five ways to begin enriching your life now:

1. Develop a can-do spirit. Feeling a sense of competence can do wonders for your self-confidence and self-esteem, as well as your quality of life. It can also give you a sense of personal control, making you feel empowered and able to tackle the challenges that lie ahead.

Push yourself intellectually by joining a reading group or taking a continuing education class. Learn a new skill or sport. Discover your hidden talents, whether it's by taking a dance or pottery class or joining a community theater group. Practice being assertive by putting your strongest foot forward in low-risk situations (at the grocery store, for instance) and gradually work up to more challenging ones.

2. Get to know yourself emotionally. All too often, women are acutely sensitive to other people's feelings but woefully out of touch with their own. It's time, then, to tap into your feelings and get to know your inner self.

Keep a mood journal and spend 5 to 10 minutes a day writing about whatever concerns you. Recognize the importance of certain relationships in your life and carve out time for them. Stop playing the self-blame game by looking for evidence that other people or factors contributed to a situation, rather than automatically taking responsibility.

continued on next page

3. Schedule personal time on a regular basis. It's important for replenishing energy and for staying in touch with who you are at heart.

Make a date with yourself to do whatever it is you want to do and pen it into your calendar and the family's calendar. Exercise good time-management skills by sticking with your priorities and trying to structure your time realistically (remember: generally, everything takes slightly longer than you think it will). Set limits with other people by being brave enough to say no (or at least "Can I get back to you?") when you're deluged with requests. Discover the benefits of solitude by spending a few moments each day just sitting quietly, reflecting on your own thoughts and feelings.

4. Cultivate a spiritual connection. This can make you feel more grounded in life and broaden your perspective on the world. Study after study has found that religiously active people experience greater happiness; this may be due to the close relationships that are engendered, to the sense of meaning and purpose people extract from their faith, and/or from the incentive people feel to extend their focus beyond themselves.

Join a church, a synagogue or another spiritual organization if the sense of community, the power of prayer, or the spiritual setting appeals to you. Bond with nature to help yourself reconnect with something in the physical, perceptible world that is much larger than you are. Help people who are in need by volunteering at a local hospital or a center for underprivileged kids.

5. Rediscover your capacity for joy. Adding more laughter and play to your life is a start but it's also important to find real contentment and satisfaction in your everyday life.

Take time to relish the small joys in life, whether it's playing tag with your kids in the backyard or appreciating the first delicate bloom on your rosebush. Introduce more humor into your life,

continued on next page

whether it's by spending time with people who make you chuckle or watching movies that make you laugh out loud. Pinpoint ways in which you may be limiting pleasure in your life—whether it's your mind-set or your schedule—and try to find new avenues for enjoyment. Learn to appreciate the present moment by breathing deeply, paying attention to your senses and letting yourself just be.

choices we actually make on any given day. We're so accustomed to making decision after decision that we often do it automatically or we simply react on instinct or impulse to the situation at hand. This tendency to go with instantaneous responses may be becoming increasingly common, given the fast-paced, high-tech times we're living in. Now that so many tasks can be achieved in the blink of an eye—e-mail correspondences sent or received, stocks bought or sold electronically—it seems as though everyone's acting like a mover and shaker. Given this frenetic pace, what many people have stopped doing is to consciously examine all the possibilities that are available to them—and consider their potential consequences.

And while we all make both good decisions and unfortunate ones from time to time, the pattern of your choices can be significant. An accumulation of good choices, for example, can bolster your self-esteem, encouraging you to make more good choices in the future and giving you the confidence to take smart risks. Repeatedly making poor choices, on the other hand, can weaken your self-esteem, which can, in turn, cause you to perpetuate a negative pattern or become skittish about making any choices in the future. For these reasons, it's important to become aware of the pattern of choices you've made in the past.

The idea isn't to make yourself pay emotionally for the choices you've made; you've already done that in some way. Besides, it's futile—and self-destructive—to beat yourself up about choices you've already made. They're history. But you can learn from them if you examine them, question your reasons for making them, and take responsibility for them. Looking back, you might ask yourself: Was buying that car a wise move or an impulsive choice? Did I accept the best job offer for me—or did I go with what felt safe? Once you begin to notice the patterns underlying your decisions, you can put yourself back in the driver's seat of your life. You can then figure out why you made a particular choice that ultimately went awry, how other options may have turned out better, and what you could do differently next time.

One of the crucial steps to take as you try to improve your life is to start making conscious choices. When you come to a point where you're faced with a decision—whether it's a minor one (Should I have this piece of chocolate cake?) or a major one (Should I invest in this mutual fund?)— try to get in the habit of building in a pause. It can be as short as ten seconds for the little decisions or as long as you need (or is reasonable, given the circumstances) for the larger ones. The point is to give yourself a substantial enough period of time to realize that the responsibility for this choice is in your hands. While you're mulling over the issue, you might ask yourself: How will I feel if I do what I'm inclined to do? What are the consequences likely to be? What might happen if I did the opposite? What would my ideal self choose to do? If you often struggle with indecisiveness, that tells you something, too—namely, that you may be out of touch with what you really want.

Above all, it's important to remember that deciding to change some aspect of yourself or your life is a choice—and it's your choice. You control the choice itself as well as the pace with which you make it. If what you're craving is immediate, dramatic change in your career, for example, you could decide to resign from your job (assuming you've weighed all the pros and cons and you've concluded that this is a smart way to go). On the other hand, if you want to ease into change, you might start setting smaller goals—such as spending one week sending out the word that you're looking for a new job, another week researching new opportunities in the library or on the Internet, another week going to informational interviews, and so on—until you feel comfortable making the leap. The point is, you're in charge of your life and you have the power to determine your destiny with every step that you take. So try to make each one count.

Honoring Yourself as a Priority

By now you probably have a fairly clear sense of your personal goals. The question is: How will you get there? It won't happen magically or automatically; you're going to have to chart your own course. The next step is to set priorities in terms of how you want to work on these goals, and then to figure out how you can address them in your life. To get the ideas flowing, get out a pen and complete the following exercise. In answer to the following questions, write down at least two sentences, even a short paragraph.

◆ What vision would you like to have of yourself in various aspects of your life, whether it's in your career, as a mother, as an athlete, or other areas?

◆ If your life were to start over tomorrow, how would you want to spend your time? What aspects of yourself that you've been neglecting would you choose to nurture?

◆ What values spur you into action? What are your core beliefs about what it means to be a good or valuable person?

◆ What do you now consider your top priorities based on what you value for your entire life? (If this question is hard for you to answer, you might consider what would be the greatest gift you could give yourself if you didn't have so many demands on your time.)

- What could you do to live in a way that's more in sync with your most cherished values and beliefs?

- What steps could you start taking to do just that—today?

After defining what's important to you, it's time to set priorities and map out your goals. Refer to your wish list from earlier in the chapter in developing these goals. Let's say you've realized that you've been neglecting your physical and emotional well-being and one of the items from your wish list is to become physically strong and fit; physical self-care should be high on your priority list. You might set specific goals to help you make that happen. For example, you might choose to dedicate 30 to 45 minutes each day to self-care, whether it's spent going to the gym, going for a walk, meditating, or taking a yoga class. If strengthening your marriage is one of your priorities, you might decide to get up half an hour earlier each morning so you can share a leisurely breakfast with your spouse before the kids arise, to plan a romantic getaway (whether it's a day or a weekend) every few months, or to cook dinner with your spouse one night a week. Similarly, if a sense of spiritual well-being has been eluding you, and you think this would help you have a more upbeat attitude toward life in general, you might choose to join a religious institution, volunteer to help those who are less fortunate in the community, or spend more time basking in nature's beauty.

Whatever items you come up with, think of this as your most valuable to-do list ever and put these activities on your calendar. From now on, this list should become a guiding force that will help you make decisions about how you choose to live. It shouldn't be a matter of finding a way to fit in these new priorities; these should be considered an essential part of improving your life. It's a subtle shift in thinking, but it will help you figure out how to handle your time differently without feeling guilty. When you recognize that these goals are an essential part of your life, it will become much easier to say no to requests that aren't meaningful (or that aren't important in the grand scheme of things) or to delegate certain responsibilities to other people. That way, you'll have the time, the space and the energy to pursue your goals.

Learning to Embrace Change

Warning: It's not necessarily going to be easy to change old habits and patterns of behavior. There's something comforting about the familiar—whether it's a physical location or a particular way of acting. The old ways may not be perfect; it may not be exciting. But they're a known, as opposed to an unknown, quantity and there's something to be said for that. At least that's how the thought process goes for many people who are resistant to—or who even go out of their way to avoid—change. They cling to their routine, making excuses for putting off challenges, for staying within their comfort zone, for making the same decisions again and again.

The nature of change requires relinquishing an aspect of the past and venturing into unknown territory. It might necessitate a shedding—or at least a readjustment—of an old self. And it certainly involves taking risks. All changes are stressful, both the happy ones (such as getting married or buying a new home) and the sad ones (such as getting divorced or moving away from beloved friends or family members). So it's unrealistic to expect that you'll feel altogether comfortable in the process of making changes.

But change can also be quite liberating. If you let yourself rise above the fear factor and picture a better way, you can then take steps to reinvent the circumstances of your life. As the American naturalist and author Henry David Thoreau once noted, "Things do not change, we do." It's up to you to assume responsibility for creating the life you want to live. Besides looking inward to assess what makes you feel happy and fulfilled, you'll need to take charge of your actions, be open-minded toward new possibilities, and make a serious commitment to pursuing your goals and dreams. No one else can take these steps for you.

ASSIGNMENT Think about how you want to live your life and write down a personal mission statement. This should reflect your philosophy of life, a statement about what kind of person you want to be and what's important to you. If you can then distill the essence of this philosophy into a catchy phrase—whether it's "Relish the moment" or "My family comes first"—you can later use this mission statement as an affirmation of what's truly important to you when you need it and as incentive to help you say no to requests that divert you from your goals and values.

CHAPTER THREE

Are You Ready to Take Charge?

People always tell me that I'm a true-to-form redhead—fiery, spontaneous and absolutely passionate about life. They are right, but there's also a side of me that's sensitive and not so sure of the world. It's this vulnerable side that I believe has always driven a need in me to please people, even when doing so doesn't make me particularly happy.

Why do I care if people like me? I think because deep in my heart I'm afraid to be completely on my own. That's how I felt when my mother re-married and moved halfway around the world when I was 12 years old. Though we always remained close and loving, her absence made me very lonely and I fumbled awkwardly through my adolescence without her sup-port. My father, a former military man, ran our home with great effi-ciency, but he was out of his league when it came to talking about dieting, body image, or dating.

Nevertheless, Dads gave our home discipline and stability, and I liked the fact that someone bigger, stronger and smarter was there for me.

I fell hard for Prince Andrew because of his self-assurance. I'd entered our marriage secure in the idea that we were an unbeatable team, but I was not prepared for the legions of help and handlers whose job it would be to man-age so much of our lives. With my husband away at sea with the Royal Navy most of the time, I quickly lost any sense of control over my own life, because I allowed so many others to take charge. I've since realized that taking control and making decisions for myself is what gives me strength and freedom.

Are you ready to take charge? If your weight is out of control I know you'll be inspired by Weight Watchers leader Sherry Fischer, who finally took the reins and started anew, scrapping her unhealthy eating habits and changing her relationship with food. Sherry's weight problem can be traced back to her childhood in Kentucky, where food was plentiful but there were few guidelines for when and how much to eat. I try to set an example for my daughters with the hope they'll be spared my problems with weight. I think it is wonderful that so many Weight Watchers members take what they learn about healthy diet and teach it to their family, because it's a gift that can last a lifetime. It has been so much fun for me to share my Weight Watchers journey with my daughters. Sometimes it's a game where they test my knowledge, as in "Mummy, how many **POINTS** for the two brownies you are about to eat?" They are great for my motivation. But beyond the humor, I think it's absolutely important to listen to my children when they speak and to honor their feelings despite their young age. I recall so clearly how, at age 12, no one listened to me when I said that I felt overweight. I needed to be heard because it all felt so confusing. I am very attentive to my girls' emotional needs because I know that learning and building confidence now will help them take charge of their lives later on.

Like me, Sherry found that the structure and discipline she learned at Weight Watchers applied to many parts of her life. You can't change everything overnight, but you can build toward a new lifestyle with small steps. Sherry says the process of change is like building up a muscle. I think she's right because you may start with nothing, but you see and feel results with every workout and soon you are stronger than ever.

Taking charge and feeling in control feels great, but let's remember to forgive ourselves for those times when we temporarily lapse into our old ways. When my mother was killed in a car crash I ate out of shock and sorrow, much as I did when she first left our home. It was a terrible time for me, and overeating caused me to gain weight as a result. I remained in control nonetheless thanks to the support of my family and my friends. Weight Watchers helped me understand why I was overeating: within a few weeks of my mother's funeral, I was back on the program and all the stronger for it.

Discovering When the Time Is Right

At first blush, it may sound counterintuitive, but growing up in a large family can foster eating habits that could be hazardous to a woman's weight. "I come from a huge family—my dad's the youngest of 19 children—so I was taught as a child to eat quickly," explains Sherry Fischer, now 47, a Weight Watchers leader in Kentucky. "Food was a big thing in my family. We always had luscious desserts and lots of everything, and we were taught to eat everything on our plates. I come from a family of big people, and I've been fluffy all my life. I think I was eight or nine when I first heard someone refer to me as overweight."

Sherry lost some weight as a teenager, and in 1970 her mother peeled off more than 100 pounds through Weight Watchers. "I was excited to see that you could eat and take weight off," recalls Sherry, a mother of two. "Before that, we thought we had to starve ourselves." Yet even though she was a witness to her mother's successful weight-loss tactics, Sherry continued to struggle with her own cycles of gaining and losing weight throughout young adulthood.

It wasn't until after the birth of her second child that Sherry decided to truly get serious about slimming down. At the age of 30, she was horrified when she caught a glimpse of herself in a picture that somebody had snapped of her in a bathing suit: Sherry had to face the fact that she was far from pleased with the shape her 5-foot 8-inch figure had assumed. "It was scary and embarrassing," she says. "It was the first time that I decided to seek help. I wanted to get the weight off and get it off healthfully." She joined Weight Watchers and within eight months took off 40 pounds.

What made this attempt more successful than all her previous ones? "Before this, I would always try to lose weight for an event—a prom, a wedding, that kind of thing," Sherry explains. "After the event was over and I'd accomplished my goal, I'd go back to what I was doing before and I'd gain the weight back. This time I wanted to do it for me. It's not enough to have willpower. You have to have want-power— and you have to be willing to do what it takes to safely get it done. I knew the time had come for me; you've got to be ready in your head and I knew I was ready this time. I woke up one morning, called to find out where the nearest Weight Watchers meeting was, and when I came in the door, I knew this was home. This was where there was hope and I knew I was going to do it when I walked through that door."

Before she could jump into the process with both feet, however, Sherry had some homework to do. "I had to make a contract with myself, a mission statement, and remove it from my head," she says. "A college professor once told me that what you hold in your head controls you; what you write down, you now have control over." So Sherry put pen to paper and wrote down her mission statement: "I want to get the weight off safely for the rest of my days on earth." She didn't set a time frame for her goal; nor did she map out step-by-step goals. That was too overwhelming to her. But she did emphasize that this time the weight would have to go—forever. "When you say you're 'losing weight,' you're always waiting for it to come home," she says. "But when you say you're removing it, it is gone for good. Weight remains removed when the process fits into who you are."

To figure out how weight removal fit into the scheme of her life, Sherry had to set priorities for losing weight, and that included drawing up short-term or daily goals. "When you set a goal, you have to consider three Rs," she says, "whether it's reasonable and realistic; if it is, it'll be reachable." With that guideline in mind, she eased into the dietary and exercise changes she wanted to make and learned to be patient with the weight-removal process, which she calls "a journey." Because Sherry is a morning person, she began taking walks around her neighborhood at 6:30 A.M. to ensure that she would exercise. Because she often craves salty, crunchy foods, she had to retrain her taste buds slightly by adjusting the characteristics of the foods she ate; she began using veggies, for example, to fulfill the need to crunch instead of gravitating toward chips and the like.

Sherry also had to become more aware of some of the negative influences in her environment and learn to handle them differently. "I had to tune out saboteurs," she admits. "I had to learn to take a stand against what other family members did at family get-togethers and reunions. You have to learn to be aggressive and to look at what works for you."

Most of all, she needed to develop consistency in her eating habits. "It was hard doing it every day," she confesses. "I had to discipline myself. Discipline is like a muscle: The more you use it, the stronger it becomes. It was a day-by-day thing. I had to be structured and stop listening to outside people. And I had to learn to forgive myself when I fell off the wagon. I had to learn from the experience and not beat myself *up for it. I didn't need to make a catastrophe out of a simple slip-up." To keep herself on course, Sherry would draw up a daily to-do list, including a plan for what she was going to eat that day. She made sure that her food scale and measuring cups were always on the counter so she wouldn't have to estimate portion sizes. "I still weigh and measure my food because guessing is what got me here in the first place," she says. "I've learned to do what works for me."*

Without a doubt, creating your own blueprint for success and giving yourself permission to use it can facilitate the quest to peel off unwanted pounds. But it's a strategy that's also relevant to the rest of a person's life. And, these days, Sherry isn't afraid to apply it. "Removing the weight taught me to be consistent and persistent in most areas of my life," she says, "because I think getting and keeping weight off is one of the hardest things to do. It gave me self-respect. It brought me here (to Weight Watchers), to a job I truly love to do. And it taught me not to be afraid to be the person that I am."

TIMING IS EVERYTHING. It's true in virtually every aspect of your life, but perhaps nowhere more so than in the process of change. Launch a plan of action when the timing is right, and you'll increase your odds of succeeding in your goals. Embark on a drive to transform yourself before you're truly ready and you may be doomed to fail, or you could lose momentum after your initial burst of enthusiasm and energy. And in case not reaching your goal isn't disappointing enough, your thwarted efforts could discourage you from trying again in the future. This can also take a toll on your self-esteem and your mood, possibly even leading you down the path to depression or anxiety.

That's why it's important to accurately assess your situation to see if you're truly ready to take charge and tackle the challenges you've set for yourself. Just because you *want* to change doesn't mean you're ready to do so. You might be talking up a blue streak about your good intentions or reading everything you can get your hands on about changing some aspect of your life or your habits, and there's nothing wrong with that as a prelude to taking action, but these aren't necessarily signs that you're ready to lose weight, change careers, leave an unhappy marriage or take steps to improve your health. And if you frequently make excuses for maintaining the status quo, if you continue to place physical or psychological obstacles in front of yourself, or if you search for miraculous tools to help you change your life, you're not in the right frame of mind to take charge, either.

Many people think that once they're armed with motivation, they will be truly ready to change. It's true that motivation is essential to the process of change, but by itself it won't make you ready to embark on the journey to altering your behavior or your life. Indeed, some psychologists believe that it's only when people are really ready to change for their own personal reasons and only when they have the willingness and the courage to deal with the emotional issues that may underlie their current behavior will they have the proper motivation and the proper mind-set to change. At that point, all kinds of different strategies can be helpful for implementing those changes. But without having a solid resolve and personally meaningful reasons for wanting to change, you're unlikely to be successful, no matter what strategies you employ.

The problem with trying to tackle major changes before you're ready is twofold. First of all, you may end up setting yourself up for failure because you're not yet willing to do what it takes to succeed. As a result, you may find yourself sabotaging your own good intentions in subtle ways or you may cave in at the earliest sign of external pressure to veer from your goals. Or you might simply resign yourself to a failed effort when the going gets tough and the challenges feel overwhelming. Second, you may wind up giving up on your desire to change—now or in the future—because it just seemed too hard to turn that desire into reality this time.

Finding the Right Stuff

So what exactly makes someone ready to embark on the challenging process of change? How can you tell if the time is truly right? First, you need to know what it is that you really want—and you have to be clear about your reasons for wanting it. If you've made these steps but your mission still isn't quite clear, you may have some more reflecting to do before you forge ahead. Next, you need to know what you are willing to do to achieve your goal. You need to be willing to take control—of your time, your environment, and your attitude, for starters—even if that means making choices that aren't always pleasant. You need to be seriously motivated for all the right reasons—namely, because *you* want to do this for *you,* not for someone else. And you need to have the sense that all your hard work and sacrifices will be worthwhile in the end.

Finally, you'll need to have an open mind, a positive attitude and a can-do spirit to help buoy your resolve when it begins to wane and to help you climb over the hurdles that lie ahead. Keeping an open mind and an upbeat outlook can also make you more receptive to helpful information that may incidentally come your way. In a recent study, researchers at the Center for Health Care Evaluation at the Veterans Affairs Palo Alto Health Care System and Stanford University found that sedentary college students who were exposed to messages about the benefits of exercise and how to initiate an exercise program were more likely to really process the information if they had an open-minded attitude; surprisingly enough, attitude turned out to be even more important than their level of intention to exercise. This is worth noting, because if there's one thing you can count on in the journey to change, it's that you'll face plenty of obstacles and you'll need to draw upon all the help you can get, both internally and externally. Some of these hurdles will be foreseeable but many won't. In either case, you may need to use flexibility in how you handle them. If one strategy doesn't work you'll need to be ready and willing to try another.

Of course, you'll also need to consider whether this is a good time in your life to embark on your particular mission. Do you have the time—or can you create the time—that it will take to pursue your goals? Is your life calm enough and sufficiently stable at the moment to be able to withstand the shock waves that making these changes might bring? If you're dealing with multiple sources of stress at the moment—a sick parent, financial strain, and intense deadlines at work, for example—it may not be prudent to invite another one right now. But if you know that these pressures will pass in a few short weeks or months, that may be a better time to launch your plans. So spend a little time thinking about whether you're ready to get going, or if you'd be better off in the long run by waiting. But also consider this: If you don't think the time is right, could you be using this as an excuse for not taking charge? And if so, what could you do to let go of this excuse and move forward?

Demystifying the Process of Change

It's not enough to want to make a change in your life, even if you feel passionate about it. And it's not enough to be clear about why you want to make this change, or to be deeply committed. To turn your best intentions into reality, it helps to understand where you are in the process of change and how you can further your progress. After all, change is a process, not an event. It begins with readiness on your part, it progresses into action, and it ends with your efforts to maintain the fruits of your labor.

In recent decades, psychologists James O. Prochaska, Carlo C. DiClemente and John C. Norcross have studied how people make lasting changes in their lives on their own. What they've found is that change typically occurs in six predictable stages and that people who push themselves to accomplish changes they're not ready for often set themselves up to fail. What these researchers and others have also discovered is that if people can pinpoint their current stage of change, they can then employ specific, effective strategies that can help push them to the next stage.

The first stage is called *precontemplation*, where a person is often resistant to change; she may be full of excuses for maintaining the status quo, or she may be giving the issue lip service in response to pressure from other people. Does this sound like you? If so, you might benefit from thinking about the self-defeating excuses that block your ability to make healthy changes in your life. Try to become conscious of when you use them and why. (For help in this area, see the section "What's Holding You Back?" on page 79.) This is also a prime time to gather information about what's involved in making the change you desire and to enlist the support of trusted friends and family members.

In the second stage, called *contemplation,* you've probably begun to think seriously about taking action but on some level you may still be struggling with internal resistance. Maybe you're waiting for the perfect time to launch your plan or maybe you're still hoping for a miracle to remove the whole issue from your life. Your best strategies, at this juncture, are to clarify why you want to change this particular aspect of your behavior or your life and what your real goals are. It's also helpful to begin monitoring your behavior. Keeping a journal can help you develop a clear picture of what your starting point is and what you should really concentrate on changing.

During the *preparation* stage, you realize that your intentions are firm and that you're on the verge of taking charge; you may even have taken baby steps toward your goal, but perhaps you haven't yet jumped into your plan with both feet. It's wise to continue to take small steps in the right direction (think of this as a warm-up to the main workout) but also to set priorities in terms of how you're going to change, and to develop a plan of action that suits your goals and your lifestyle. To do this, it may help to gather advice from other people who've tackled similar challenges.

During these initial stages, it's crucial to assess whether you're truly ready to take charge and really strive for your goal. Why? Because otherwise you're likely to get stuck in your efforts, which could cause you to become frustrated and give up. Next comes the *action stage,* where it's time to hatch your plan for transforming your habits or your life; the *maintenance* phase, where the challenge is to make these changes permanent; and, finally, the *termination stage,* at which point you've completely changed your behavior. You'll read more about these phases in later chapters.

Is Your Head in the Right Place?

Before you push yourself to get going, identify your starting point by assessing whether you have the right stuff to go forth and take charge. You can find out by taking this quiz. Read the following statements and mark them True or False as they pertain to you.

1. I've given a lot of thought to the specific steps I'll need to take to achieve my goal.

2. I recognize some of the challenges and roadblocks that may lie ahead and I've thought about how I might handle them.
3. I've decided to pursue this change now because I really want to, not because someone else has pressured me to.
4. My life is unusually stressful at the moment but I've decided that this is as good a time as any to get started with this plan.
5. I'm prepared to commit a reasonable amount of time and effort every week to pursuing these goals.
6. I want this dream to come true but I'm not sure I'll be able to sustain motivation if it takes a long time.
7. I've identified personal strengths I can rely on along the way.
8. I've given myself a hard-and-fast deadline within which I should reach my goal.
9. I want to launch my plan of action now even though my emotions have been on a roller coaster lately.
10. I suspect that making these changes is going to be difficult but I believe that I have the mental toughness and stamina to deal with the rigors that are involved.
11. I've tried to achieve this goal before and I hope I'll be more successful this time, but I can't be sure that I will be.
12. I expect to feel like a different person once I've achieved my goal.

SCORING: Tally up your responses. There is no ideal score, but the higher your total is (a maximum of 24 is possible), the greater your chances of being successful if you pursue your plan now. But don't worry if your score is lower than you'd like it to be. Simply read the corresponding explanations in the following pages to see where your mind-set may be amiss on a particular question. Once you've done that, you can work on giving your attitude an adjustment.

1. T: 2, F: 1   *2.* T: 2, F: 1   *3.* T: 2, F: 1   *4.* T: 1, F: 2   *5.* T: 2, F: 1
6. T: 1, F: 2   *7.* T: 2, F: 1   *8.* T: 1, F: 2   *9.* T: 1, F: 2   *10.* T: 2, F: 1
11. T: 1, F: 2   *12.* T: 1, F: 2

1. The importance of thinking ahead: When you gain an understanding of what it takes to change a habit or achieve a certain goal, you make the undertaking that much easier on yourself. Why? Because you've made an effort to anticipate what's involved and to plan ahead. This helps to bridge the gap between good intentions and effective action.

2. Why it's smart to anticipate roadblocks: When you envision potential challenges that may come up, you'll find them much less jarring when you actually encounter them. This is a form of mental rehearsal, and it can help prepare your mind and body to deal with a situation in a way that will further your progress toward your goal.

3. Why do it for yourself: To be successful in your endeavor, the desire and commitment have to come from you. You have to take responsibility for the choices you make. Friends and family can help you by providing support and encouragement along the way, but it's not healthy for someone else to be your motivating force. After all, you're the one who's going to be doing all the work.

4. The wisdom of choosing a calm climate: Embarking on a major change when life is already stressful is adding insult to injury. It might also be considered self-sabotaging behavior, because emotional upheaval can undermine your resolve to stick with your plan. You'd be better off waiting to set sail on a calmer day.

5. The importance of parceling out time: It's smart and realistic to plan to devote a certain amount of time each day and each week to pursuing your goals. It's even a good idea to mark it in your calendar and to treat it as a sacred appointment. This way, you'll minimize the chances of other demands interfering with this priority.

6. Why you need enduring motivation: If you have doubts about being able to sustain motivation from the beginning, you could be headed for trouble. After all, plenty of challenges will arise along the way that will test how truly motivated you are. If your motivation is shaky to begin with, you'd be wise to shore it up before moving forward.

7. The benefits of assessing your strengths: You're going to need your strengths and your resourcefulness when the going gets tough, so it's a good idea to know where they lie ahead of time. That way, when you're faced with a challenge, you can simply turn inward for support and sustenance.

8. Why it's good to be flexible: It's fine to attach a time frame to your goal, but the ability to bend and adjust is important. Otherwise, you could be setting yourself up for a huge disappointment—not to mention a setback if the window of opportunity you've allowed turns out to be unrealistic. Research has found that people who fail often think they've changed their ways within a short period of time, when, in fact, it can take three to six months to get a new pattern established and even longer to really make it part of your life.

9. Why seizing the moment isn't always smart: That old saying "There's no time like the present" is helpful when it comes to preventing yourself from procrastinating. But it's not altogether prudent if you're planning to embark on a major change while you're dealing with emotional stresses and strains. You'll be making life extremely difficult for yourself, which isn't exactly helpful when you're trying to alter your life.

10. The importance of mental vigor: When it comes to changing your behavior, a sense of self-efficacy—a belief that you have the will and the way to achieve your goals—is a powerful force indeed. Study after study has found this to be true—and it likely will be for you.

11. The wisdom of learning from the past: Previous failures are nothing to be ashamed of. But unless you've learned from them and used them to strengthen your resolve for the next attempt, you're not doing much to bolster your chances of success the next time around.

12. Why you shouldn't set unrealistic expectations: Once you achieve your goal, you very well might feel like a different person, but this is just as likely to be a result of enduring the process as achieving the result. Besides, achieving your goal should be its own reward.

Now that you've completed this quiz, you probably have a keener sense of whether you're ready to make long-term changes. The idea isn't to make a decision based solely on the results of this self-assessment but to use it to help you consider the concept of readiness and how it applies to you. By exploring these possibilities before forging ahead, you'll be doing yourself a favor. The very idea that you could want something badly and intend to make it happen but not be quite ready to do so is a foreign concept to many people. So just by considering change, you'll gain a clearer perspective on your mind-set and attitude, as well as on the facts of your life and how they could help or hinder you in your efforts. After all, change doesn't happen in a vacuum. The cold, hard truth is: Making any significant change in your life requires considerable time and effort on your part if the result is going to be successful. You can follow lots of different plans and consult various guides, such as this one, to help you navigate the road to change. But in the end, completing the journey is truly up to you and you alone.

Do a Cost-Benefit Analysis

When it comes to making significant changes in behavior, weighing the benefits against the drawbacks or sacrifices that are involved can help determine if you're ready to take action. If you'd like to lose weight, for example, you might consider the benefits—such as improved health, more energy, being able to look more attractive (or whatever matters to you personally). Then compare them with the potential downsides—you might feel hungrier than usual, your new eating plan may be difficult and time-consuming to implement, you may have to give up your favorite foods. Likewise, if you want to quit smoking, you might weigh the pros of kicking the habit—improved health, an increased life span, breathing easier, no longer smelling like smoke—against the constant unpleasant withdrawal symptoms and cravings and possible weight gain. Similarly, if you want to find a more challenging job, the benefits might include increased psychic satisfaction, greater résumé-building potential, increased opportunities for promotion and greater earning power. The drawbacks, on the other hand, might include the time-consuming aspect of actually looking for a job, the stress of readjusting to a new environment, and giving up the camaraderie of your current situation.

Whatever your goal may be, write a list of *all* the potential benefits and drawbacks of making this change on a piece of paper or in your journal. In constructing this list, consider how making this change might affect your physical and emotional well-being, your social environment, your personal growth, your time (including your leisure hours), your relationships with family and friends, your career and your overall quality of life.

Once you've drawn up your lists, mark whether each item applies in the long term or only in the short term. For example, improved health is a long-term benefit of both losing weight and giving up smoking, whereas feeling hungrier than usual and dealing with unpleasant withdrawal symptoms are both short-term drawbacks. This exercise can help you see how the benefits and drawbacks stack up against each other. Gaining this perspective may even tip the balance in one direction, helping you decide if you're ready to take charge of this endeavor.

Don't be surprised if some unpleasant emotions surface in the course of performing this exercise: You might feel anxious about the future, insecure about the present, or regretful about the past. Although these feelings can be unsettling, they are a natural part of the process and you can use them to your advantage. In fact, when researchers at the University of Washington in Seattle evaluated the effect of enhancing personal awareness of the negative consequences of substance use (alcohol, cigarettes and the like) on readiness to change, they found that regret seemed to play an important role in the decision to change. In another study, researchers at the University of Washington in Seattle found that focusing on specific losses that are related to substance abuse helped people gain sufficient motivation to be ready to change their ways. This strategy could even be helpful in assessing readiness to make other changes such as losing weight or starting a new career. Noting the losses you've incurred as a result of maintaining the status quo—not being able to play actively with your young kids if you're overweight, for example, or not having the intellectual stimulation you crave if you've been stuck in a ho-hum job—can also help you muster the courage to make a change.

And yet most people don't use regret that way. They simply feel sad about what they've lost or about the mistakes they've made, and they leave it at that. But by its nature, regret holds valuable information: It can tell you what you've been missing from your life and, as a result, what really matters to you. It can tell you that you should have handled a situation differently than you did. In many cases, although you can't do anything to change the past, you *can* learn from your own history and use this knowledge to create a better future for yourself. The more reasons you have for pursuing a goal and the stronger your commitment is to reaching it, the more likely you will be to maintain motivation and comply with the plan you set for yourself. And that means your chances of succeeding will be stronger.

Getting Behind the Wheel

The timing for making the changes you crave is up to you. It's not a matter of reading the tea leaves or consulting a crystal ball, or looking to any other external guide. You'll need to rely on your feelings, attitudes and intuition to tell you whether you should move forward. Take a close look at your internal barometer and see what it tells you. If the answer is no, you're not ready, don't be too discouraged. There's actually some good news: Having gone through this self-exploration exercise, you're in a better position to recognize when the time is truly right for you to take charge.

And if you're not quite ready but you're close, you can take steps now to nudge yourself in the right direction. By this point, you've probably gained some insights into the areas where you could boost your readiness, perhaps by becoming clearer about what's motivating you, by taking steps to make your emotional life more balanced, or by formulating goals that are more realistic given your circumstances. Once you've laid the groundwork, you'll put yourself in a much better starting place when you do begin your journey to change. And if you're still unsure about whether you should tackle your goals at this particular time, why not do a test run? Instead of putting off your efforts, take some small steps in the right direction. Try doing one thing differently in the area you want to change and see how it feels. If you want to lose weight, you might stop cooking with butter and start using a nonstick cooking spray instead; if you're interested in launching a new career, consider taking a class in that field (perhaps in the evenings or over a weekend) to get an inside perspective. If you like the experience, embrace it and move forward. If you're still not sure, you might test the waters a little longer.

After all, being truly ready and willing to change is half the battle. There's no denying that changing your ways is difficult. We're all creatures of habit, and old habits are hard to shake. So you'll need to have a healthy sense of self-esteem, a fair amount of mental vigor, a deep reservoir of motivation, and a strong foundation of commitment to weather the storms you'll inevitably encounter on the road to change. By bolstering your resolve, and by putting your unfinished mental and emotional business in order ahead of time, you'll improve your chances of success whenever you do take charge. The reality is, it's much easier to build your dream house on a solid foundation than a shaky one.

What's Holding You Back?

As a woman, your plate of responsibilities is probably overflowing to begin with, between working, coordinating family schedules, keeping the household running smoothly, taking care of family members and friends, and having a semblance of a life. But if you think that all this has stopped you from making meaningful changes, look below the surface at the obstacles that may be preventing you from pursuing your goals. In the end, you're really only shortchanging yourself of a better you and a better quality of life. Here are eight factors that often prevent people from being ready to pursue the changes they crave:

Fear.

It's an instinct that's essential for survival because it triggers the fight-or-flight response, prompting you to do whatever it takes to fight for your life or run as fast as you can to get away from danger. But fear can also stand in your way of achieving your goals and dreams. You could be using it, perhaps without realizing that you are, to rationalize maintaining the status quo (by thinking, "Making this change is just too scary"). Or you could be using it, unconsciously, to avoid recognizing what you need to do to effect change (instead of taking the hard road that's likely to lead to success, you take the easy way, which may not). Or you could be using fear to protect yourself from trying something again if it didn't work the first time ("Why should I put myself through the pain of failing again?"). Whichever way fear may be guiding your decisions, it's likely holding you back because it's allowing you to seek comfort in the familiar, even if it's not ultimately in your best interest. You'll need to try to get past your fears—by using relaxation techniques and by giving yourself pep talks. Remind yourself that it's okay to be afraid or apprehensive, but that fear alone isn't a good enough reason not to try something that's worthwhile.

Previous failures.

If you've tried before to tackle the goals that you've set for yourself, you may feel somewhat discouraged about making another attempt. After all, failing at something can take a toll on your self-esteem and your mood, which can make trying again that much harder. But it really depends on how you look at past attempts: Rather than viewing an unsuccessful attempt as a failure or a sign of a lack of willpower, consider it a learning experience that holds valuable lessons. If you evaluate what went wrong and what you could do differently the next time around, you'll increase your chances of success when you do try again. At that point, what's really important is to find special things you can do for yourself to prevent yourself from becoming easily discouraged or from giving up. In a study of New Year's resolutions, researchers at the University of Scranton discovered that people who successfully changed their ways had the same number of slips as their unsuccessful counterparts during the first month, but the successful people forged ahead. The secret is to be willing to try again wholeheartedly and to try doing things differently next time.

Ambivalence.

You might think you'd know if you were ambivalent about making a change. But sometimes these mixed feelings can be deeply buried, in which case they might affect your behavior while you think your motivation is intact. For instance, you might think that you want to land a more challenging job, but if you continuously but subtly sabotage your chances of doing so in interviews, that's a sign that you may want to think twice about what you really want. Similarly, if you believe that you want to adopt healthier eating habits and lose weight but you find yourself undermining your own goals by snacking around the clock, you might question what's really going on. Maybe you're afraid of what could happen (you might gain the courage to leave an unhappy marriage, you might attract more physical attention, or whatever you might be worried about) if you actually achieve those goals.

If your behavior begins to send you clues that you may have ambivalent feelings about making the changes you think you want to make, you'll need to evaluate what may be preventing you from pursuing your goals effectively. Also, consider the possibility that your ambivalence could stem from a conflict between short-term sacrifice (or short-term satisfaction) and the long-term advantages: You want to be able to enjoy that piece of cake right now, for example, but you want to lose weight over the long haul. Either way, it's important to examine your conflicting feelings and to deal with them. Otherwise, you'll just be setting yourself up for an impossible task: working against yourself instead of with yourself.

Feelings of helplessness.

In many ways, it's easier to let yourself feel like a victim of circumstances or to blame other people for what's happened in the past than to seize control over your life. This way, action isn't called for; you can just sit back and let things happen to you. But they aren't likely to turn out the way you want them to. Inertia is a close cousin to helplessness, as well as procrastination and apathy. If you're not careful, the more you give in to it, the more likely it is to take over your life and you'll *really* feel stuck in a rut. The truth is, helplessness is often a learned response: It's a reaction to events that may seem to be out of your control, and it may have been developed when you were young, but it can be unlearned. It will take a considerable amount of effort, though. This isn't to say that everything that happens to you is within your control. On the contrary, things may have happened to you, particularly when you were a child, over which you had no control. There's no reason even to consider trying to take responsibility for those events; but you should try to put them where they belong—in the past—rather than letting them dictate how you respond to current and future events. Then, too, some things that happen in the future will be beyond your control—if your home is burglarized, for example. But many challenges in your life—applying for a new job, finding a new home, reconciling with an estranged friend, among others—are within your control *if* you choose to take control. When you begin to realize that you can take the wheel and steer your own life, you'll begin to break the patterns of helplessness.

Procrastination.

For many people, putting off today what can be done tomorrow comes naturally. The trouble is, when it comes to doing anything optional, tomorrow never comes. As a result, they just keep delaying the start of their journey toward change. Procrastination can take many forms, but among the most common are postponing activities that should be a priority and giving a halfhearted effort instead of a full-fledged one because you've created a time crunch for yourself. But fear or ambivalence can also be at the heart of procrastination. You might be afraid of failing when you try to take giant steps toward self-improvement; or you might feel ambivalent about making the commitment to taking those steps because it seems too difficult, too time-consuming, too scary. The prescription for procrastination: adopt the mantra "Just do it now!" Set your priorities, schedule a reasonable block of time in which to complete them, make a firm commitment to do this, be organized and be persistent, and follow through. Once you take the first crucial step to launch your plan of action, your momentum will often carry you forward.

Perfectionism.

Warning: This form of all-or-nothing thinking is hazardous to personal progress. Why? Because it sets standards that are unrealistically high and impossible to attain. Because it tends to make you regard anything short of perfection—which is really just an illusion—as unacceptable, which can lead to anger, impatience, frustration and depression. As a result, you'll never be satisfied with your endeavors because the end result will never be good enough (i.e., perfect). So you might suffer a setback when the outcome isn't perfect or you might figure, Why bother to try if I can't do it perfectly? After a while, your innate desire for self-preservation might kick in and prevent you from even trying to achieve some of the goals you'd like to reach. But the trouble isn't with the effort but with the goals or standards you've set. The solution: Forget about trying to be perfect; instead, strive for excellence in what you do. At the same time, learn to give yourself a break when things don't turn out as you'd planned. How? By trying to identify your perfectionistic thoughts and countering them with realistic alternatives. For example, if you're upset that the cake you made for your son's birthday party didn't come out the way you'd hoped, your natural inclination might be to consider yourself a lousy mother for botching his big day; what you should point out to yourself, instead, is that your son and all his friends had a blast at the party, which was really the goal to begin with.

Misconceptions about what's actually involved.

You may be harboring some erroneous perceptions about what it takes to achieve your goal. One way to give yourself a reality check is to keep a record of exactly what you're doing now in whatever area you want to change—whether it's your diet, your exercise habits, or your job status. Once you have a clear picture of what's really going on, you can start by making whatever change you think would be easiest. If you've been thinking that it's just too difficult to revamp your eating habits, you could begin by cutting out one high-fat food or trying a new fruit or vegetable every other day. Likewise, if the idea of searching for a new job seems too daunting, you could ease into it by sending out three résumés a week. Visualize yourself making that change and it'll be easier to turn into a regular practice. Making changes doesn't have to be as hard as people often make it out to be; you can do it at your own pace and in your style. The key is to just start to do one thing to bring yourself closer to your goal.

Perceived roadblocks.

"I'm in such a perpetual time crunch that it's hard for me to . . . (fill in the blank—exercise, eat right, send out résumés, spend more time with my spouse)." "I don't have enough energy to pursue these goals." "Spending all this time on myself makes me feel guilty or selfish." Do any of these lines sound familiar? If so, you're using excuses to justify what you've chosen to do. There may not be anything real standing in your way of making progress, which means that these justifications should signal you to start trying to overcome the barriers in your head. How? By making a list of what you think is blocking your path to change and then countering each roadblock with a possible way around it. For example, if you're not making the time to exercise because you're in a constant time crunch, try looking for new opportunities to fit in movement—for example, by working out with a friend instead of meeting for lunch. You can find workable solutions; you might just need to be creative about it.

ASSIGNMENT Explore whether this is the time to push yourself to make the changes you hunger for by making a list of excuses that have stood in the way of pursuing your dream. Keep in mind that these are basically self-limiting beliefs that you've been applying to yourself unfairly. So it's time for a reality check. Next to each excuse, write down at least one reason why that excuse may be inaccurate or invalid. Next to that, jot down an empowering thought, such as "I deserve to make this happen" or "I can do this," that could help propel you over that hurdle. Now that you've countered all the excuses that have prevented you from moving forward, do you feel that you can forge ahead? If so, go for it.

CHAPTER FOUR

How to Motivate Yourself to Change

Y ou may think I'm a bit mad, but I have a little voice that speaks to me. I call her my private Sarah, because she really is my true voice, the real me. My private Sarah's only recently come back after being away for a long time. Now I can't imagine my life without her because she's become such a dear confidante and friend. There was a time when I treated my inner Sarah horribly with a constant barrage of criticism for not measuring up, and after a while, I finally drove her deep into hiding. When my life unraveled and I was truly alone, I was empty without her humor, compassion, honesty and loyalty. I needed her more than ever.

If your inner voice has gone quiet, I assure you that you can bring it back, just as I did. For me this happened when I was losing weight because the journey reawakened corners of myself where I found extraordinary reserves of truth, strength and inspiration. I'd always been athletic and a fearless competitor; I tapped into that spirit as I set out to get physically active again. My eye for color and design took new delight in finding clothes that made me look and feel attractive. My deep pride and profound love for my girls proved an enormous source of inspiration for me. Finding truth in my heart brought many intense feelings as I got control over my body, and by channeling them I was able achieve my goal.

In this next chapter you'll meet Weight Watchers leader Andrea Nishan, who discovered a whole new side of herself when she decided to lose weight. Like me, Andrea was a comfort eater and not someone who liked to exercise. She'd been heavy as a child and she was haunted by bad feelings about her body. Though Andrea had dieted plenty of times before, it wasn't until she became a Weight Watchers member that she finally learned how to set realistic goals for herself and then track a steady path to achieve them.

What I find so interesting about Weight Watchers is that the process really helps you recognize the feelings that trigger you to overeat. A real breakthrough for me was learning to reinterpret my binge trigger as a symptom of something unrelated to food that was bothering me. For example, I still sometimes feel the urge to overeat right before taking a trip abroad, but now I understand that it's a signal that I'm fearful about leaving my girls. Now, instead of overeating, I give them each a great big hug.

Lately, I've been making a concerted effort not to take the things that happen in life so personally. While on vacation this past summer, for example, I was confronted with a situation where a close friend suddenly began giving me the cold shoulder, and I immediately concluded that I had done something wrong. I began falling into my bad habits, trying to please her and to convince her to like me again. And then it struck me: Why am I taking this so personally? Why shouldn't I trust my inner voice and consider the possibility that perhaps none of this had been my fault in the first place and that the problem could very well have been hers and not mine at all? I really grew from that experience. Now I don't rush to blame myself for others' actions and I'm more willing to let go if necessary because I know in my heart that I can't please everybody all the time. "Cut loose Mother Goose," as we used to say when I was a schoolgirl.

Andrea's defeatist attitude had always stood in the way of her losing weight. Going to Weight Watchers allowed her to recognize her "inner critic" and substitute positive self-talk to dispel years of negativity and self-doubt. She told me that learning to recognize and act on her true feelings gave her an amazing sense of being in control. By acting on what really mattered to her, what I call living in truth, Andrea uncovered an incredible repository of pure inspiration.

Profile: ANDREA NISHAN
Keeping My Eyes on the Prizes

For as long as Andrea Nishan can remember, food was offered as an expression of comfort and affection in her family. "My parents fed me constantly; they used food to show love," she recalls. "I'd go around the corner to get ice cream every day. And I grew up with the clean plate club—at home and at parochial school, where someone stood over you to make sure you finished what was on your plate. I was always overweight, even as a child. In those days, you were considered healthy if you were chubby."

Though she'd tried to lose weight before, she successfully lost—and kept off— 60 pounds after joining Weight Watchers in 1981. What made this time different? "I really wanted it this time," says Andrea, now 49, a mother of two in Massachusetts. "I had four friends doing it with me. There was a little healthy competition between us, but we also had quite a nice support group. We'd take turns preparing the Weight Watchers recipes and we'd go back to one friend's house after a meeting for a meal and have our own meeting. I learned to plan my meals carefully, and I used a lot more discipline than I'd ever dreamed I had. I stayed as busy as I could to distract myself from eating; I'd go out for a walk or just find some way to get out of the house. I also made sure I wasn't alone when I cleaned up after meals—sometimes I'd ask my daughter to stay with me—so I wouldn't eat what was left on other people's plates. Once I started losing weight, it felt good to hear compliments from other people. I never had those before."

Within seven months, Andrea had reached her goal weight. Two years later, she became a Weight Watchers leader and an ambassador. Along with the help of her friends, Andrea credits continuous goal setting as the secret to her weight-loss success. "I set goals all the time to keep me motivated," she confesses. "And every time I meet one, I set another one. For example, even now, I put stars on my calendar every day that I exercise, and at the end of the month, I want to see more stars than not. I don't like to exercise, but I walk three to four times a week, and the star system keeps me going. Every fall and winter, I take out an old pair of black pants just to see how they fit. They're so old that they're shiny. My goal is just to fit into them each year, and I have for 19 years."

In addition, she kept a journal while trying to lose weight. "I'd write down everything I ate. My policy is: If you bite it, you write it—and I'd file weeks' worth of menus," she recalls. "If I got bored on the plan, I'd look back in the file and redo a week that really worked for me." To this day, Andrea continues to bargain or make deals with herself to stay on track. "I love Diet Coke," she confesses. "But before I can have a Diet Coke, I have to drink 32 ounces of water—and I do this every day. There are some days when I don't get the Diet Coke. I also believe my body works well if I eat fish several times a week, so I set a goal of eating fish three times a week." What's more, Andrea looks to the future for motivation. She often uses events—such as family reunions or anniversaries—for incentive to keep up the healthy eating and exercise habits that help her to stay slim. "If I don't have an event to look forward to, I'll throw a party," she says. "I constantly play games with myself to stay motivated."

Why go to so much trouble? "It's easy to get tired and to not want to do this anymore," she explains. "When you do this day in and day out, it's easy to slip back. I know I can go back there, to regaining the weight, and I don't want to. But I have a choice—I can stop doing what I'm doing and gain the weight back. Or I can continue to do this and win. If you don't have goals, you don't have anything to keep you going. It has to become a lifestyle change."

Over the years, as she's made this lifestyle change, Andrea has also focused on adjusting her attitude in a positive direction. "Attitude is everything," she says. "You've got to look at what you can do, not what you can't. If you believe you can do something, you really can. It's just not as fast as everyone wants. Losing weight really helped my attitude. I've grown so much. I have a saying—that if you always do what you always did, you'll always get what you always got. That saying helps me take chances, and I'm not afraid to make mistakes anymore.

"When you lose weight, you learn to take chances and put yourself out there," says Andrea, who got divorced several years ago and married a fellow Weight Watchers member in 1999. ("He always says he's the only one who went to Weight Watchers and gained 100 pounds because he got the leader," Andrea says, laughing.) "My self-esteem is so much better now. I used to be quiet; I was shy. Now I could do Carnegie Hall. When you have confidence in yourself, you don't mind trying new things because you're not afraid to fail. This attitude has helped me in the workforce—I've even talked my way into jobs—and I don't ever feel alone now. I can go anywhere and strike up a conversation with strangers."

Along with this burgeoning sense of self-confidence, Andrea discovered that her energy level soared as a result of losing weight. "I had no idea my energy level would change," admits Andrea, who is 5 feet 2 inches. "Now my activity level is extremely high. I wake up raring to go and I'm on the go all day long. There's more excitement in your life when you can do more.

"Weight loss can be a great ride if you learn from it," she adds. "You can learn a lot about yourself, about your strengths. After losing weight, I'm stronger and I'm able to put myself first—or at least on the list—without any guilt. I feel that everyone benefits if I take time for myself and do things for myself. I've learned that it's okay to be your own best friend."

FOR MANY PEOPLE, motivation is like a fickle lover—hot then cold, capricious or flighty. It often has a here-today-gone-tomorrow quality and carries with it an enthusiasm that waxes and wanes. That's because many people have a faulty impression of what it takes to be truly and effectively motivated; as a result, they tend to rely on the wrong stuff. More often than not, they think it comes from some *thing* (perhaps a structured plan or an upcoming event) or some*one* (a skilled career coach, a personal trainer, or a weight-loss counselor). They look to these external forces to provide them with the incentive and the sustenance they need to reach their goals.

But the truth is, self-motivation, the kind that originates from within, is the best spark to achieving lasting change. Why? Because it's like giving your goal a personal endorsement, according to Edward L. Deci, Ph.D., a professor of psychology at the University of Rochester. Internal or self-motivation comes from a person's deciding that she is ready to take responsibility for managing herself. It comes from a strong desire to change for herself rather than for someone else. It comes from an internal drive that generates enthusiasm, passion, commitment and perseverance in a particular course of action. And it comes from formulating a game plan that will bring you closer to personally meaningful desires.

Motivation, Part One: External

One of the latest theories about how to successfully maintain motivation revolves around the concept that there are two types of motivation: external and internal.

External motivation, or doing something simply as a means to an end, can bring about changes in behavior in the short term. But this shift is often temporary because the motivating factor is about gaining a reward or avoiding some sort of punishment. Even if the change in behavior is sustained, achieving success can sometimes feel hollow because you've gone after it for the wrong reasons. Perhaps the biggest problem with external motivation is that it often can't serve as a guiding force because it lacks personal meaning. When you consider this, it's no wonder that a study at the University of Rochester found that aspiring for financial success purely for material reasons—rather than for personally relevant ones—was associated with lower emotional well-being and more behavioral disorders.

What's more, pursuing a goal simply to comply with somebody else's ideas or popular images, which are both forms of external motivation, is also risky. In these instances, people decide to alter their ways because other people are pressuring them to or because they think they should based on what they've been told (about how to live longer or get ahead in business, for example) or because they want to conform to a certain image. The trouble is, what often comes with compliance is its polar opposite, defiance—the urge to rebel, sooner or later, against what somebody else has told you that you should be doing. Let's say the only reason you've decided to lose weight is because your spouse wants to show you off at his college reunion. If you wind up struggling with the weight-loss process, you could decide to bail out of the pursuit entirely and wind up resenting him for pushing you to do something you didn't really want to do in the first place; or, worse, you might rebel by overeating, and thus gain weight. Either way, you'd be in a lose-lose situation.

Motivation Tips and Tricks

It's true that motivation should come from the inside out. But there are a variety of strategies you can use to sustain your motivation or to jump-start it when it wanes. Many of these originate from within because they stem from your vision of what it means to be successful. You can turn to these whenever you hit a plateau in your efforts, whenever you feel like throwing in the towel, or whenever your goal seems to be such a faint glimmer on the horizon that you're beginning to wonder if it's a mirage.

Visualize excellence. Picture exactly what you want to happen, whether it's you delivering a flawless speech before your colleagues, sprinting across the finish line in a running race, or acing a professional exam. If you imagine yourself performing at your peak and you use all of your senses to create a vivid picture, you'll experience a taste of your ultimate goal.

Shake up your routine. When you begin to feel like you're taking the same steps over and over again, it's time to present yourself with a new challenge. It could be trying a new form of exercise if you're trying to get in shape or attending a professional seminar if you're trying to jump-start a stalled career.

Find inspiring role models. Take note of someone or a few people whose style, energy and commitment to their goals you really admire. Watch those people in action and talk to them about how they sustain their motivation. Then borrow or steal their strategies—shamelessly!—and bring these people to mind for inspiration when you need it.

Repeat an energizing mantra. Silently (or at least quietly) saying something as simple as "I can do this!" can serve as a powerful reminder that you have the will and the way to succeed. Using affir-

continued on next page

mations in this manner is a form of positive self-talk, and it can help pump you up with the vitality and mental vigor you need to keep going when you feel like quitting.

Remember a time when you were overflowing with a can-do spirit. Reflect back on a time in your life when you felt so driven to succeed that nothing could possibly stop you. Recall how energized your mind and body felt, how amazingly in control you seemed to be. Then try to recapture that feeling in your behavior. Walk, talk and act as if you actually feel full of motivation and confidence now.

Become the great impersonator. When your motivation leaves you high and dry and you feel absolutely stuck, take a break from your style and act like someone you admire. It might be a matter of pretending you are your boss's supervisor, who is a compelling public speaker, when you need to give a presentation, or acting like an athlete you admire when you need mental and physical vigor for a daunting exercise challenge.

Imagine your frustration going up in smoke. Picture the frustration leaving your body—and, most important, your mind—and envision new energy taking its place. If you can picture this happening in your mind's eye, the odds are it'll give you the energy and enthusiasm you need to persevere. After all, seeing is believing.

Give yourself a mental vacation. Sometimes pursuing a goal day after day can wear you out emotionally. This isn't surprising when you consider that change is stressful, even if it will ultimately turn out to be a positive form of stress. If these other strategies don't relieve mental malaise, give yourself a day—or even a week—off from your plan. This may be just what you need to replenish motivation and get you back on track again.

Motivation, Part Two: Internal

Internal motivation is the energy that's produced and sustained by the positive emotions you feel as you go about pursuing your goal. Not surprisingly, a significant body of research has found that internal or self-motivation is far likelier to lead to positive emotions and health-promoting behaviors than motivation that is controlled by external factors.

Internal motivation is comprised of four elements: *choice, purpose, mastery,* and *progress.* It begins with your *choosing* your goals, progresses to your embracing a *purpose*, evolves as you gain a sense of *mastery* from your hard work, and continues to bloom if you allow yourself to enjoy the *progress* and milestones you reach along the way.

Let's look at these components more closely. It's important to remember that it's been your choice to tackle this project, and the ability to maintain a feeling of autonomy—the feeling that you're taking these steps because you want to, not because you have to or should—helps you choose how you will pursue your goal. This freedom of choice can help spark your motivation to begin with (because you decided to embark on this challenge) as well as sustain motivation along the way (because you always have the option of abandoning this mission).

One of the other essential ingredients for internal motivation is to have a sense of purpose, a guiding force. It's right there inside you; you just need to unearth your sense of purpose and nurture it. And when it no longer suits your life? You can reinvent it (when you decide to make a career change, for example, or when suddenly you've got an empty nest and it's time to figure out the next step in your life). Then your challenge is to develop a *new* sense of purpose to give your life direction, substance and spirit. Not only does this sense of purpose serve as an internal compass that guides your behavior, but you can also draw on it as from a deep well of meaning. It can even buffer you from stress; in fact, a study from Brock University in Canada found that teachers and school administrators who had strong internal work values—which can provide a sense of purpose— were less likely to be affected by stress than those who lacked such values.

Moreover, having an ongoing impression that what you are doing is worthwhile, valuable or important in some way acts as motivation and empowerment to continue to do whatever it is you are doing. It's rather like the feeling you'd get if you were on an adventure with a mission: You'd feel that you were in pursuit of something that was worth your time and energy, that all your efforts would somehow pay off in the eventual scheme of things, no matter how challenging the journey turned out to be.

Of course, as you give your best effort to pursuing your mission, you can take pride in the fact that you've mastered something and are doing it. With every milestone that you reach, your sense of competence will rise a notch or two; after all, feeling competent reflects being able to meet an optimal challenge. This sense of mastery can enhance your self-esteem. Indeed, in a study at Southern Utah University, researchers found that college students who were internally motivated to exercise experienced more of the mood-boosting effects that are associated with physical activity than those who were externally motivated; the internally motivated group also gained a greater sense of competence and satisfaction from exercising than the other group did. There's no denying that feeling good— or better—about yourself is a powerful reward, and it's an addictive one at that: It makes you want to put your best foot forward and take smart risks, which can help you expand your comfort zone and boost your self-esteem even more. These built-in psychological rewards make you want to progress even further—and keep striving . . . and striving.

The final component of internal motivation comes into play as you're advancing toward your goal. It simply *feels good*—that is, if you let yourself pay attention to your progress. Unfortunately, many people keep their eyes so closely trained on the ultimate prize that they miss all the smaller payoffs along the way to their goal. This short-sighted approach is detrimental for three reasons: One, they're less likely to enjoy the process; two, they're robbing themselves of built-in sources of satisfaction; and, three, they're straining their motivation by not allowing it to be naturally buoyed by the inherent rewards of progress. Don't fall into this trap; enjoy the journey as well as the destination.

Striking a Balance

While it's best to be internally motivated to pursue a goal, there's no reason that you can't use external rewards to keep yourself going. It's not wise to rely *solely* on external rewards, but you can use a combination of naturally occurring internal rewards and self-created external ones to sustain motivation over the long haul. The idea isn't to use external rewards to control your own behavior but to promote and reinforce some of the constructive changes you've begun to make.

Before you can tap into any form of motivation, however, you'll need to come up with a plan. The first step is to pinpoint what your goals are and why they are important to you or what you hope to get from reaching them. Don't gloss over this point: This is really the crux of the issue because it's only when you imbue your goals with a sense of personal meaning that you can begin to think about what's going to motivate you. (You'll learn more about the keys to effective goal setting in Chapter 6.) But there's also a "Which comes first, the chicken or the egg?" element at work here since motivation comes naturally when you pursue meaningful goals for personally significant reasons. Letting motivation grow from the ground up is an organic process; simply put, the effort becomes a labor of love.

Striving for change is an area where you just can't fake motivation. If you aren't really hungry for the goals you've set for yourself, nothing outside you will jump-start your motivation sufficiently. Otherwise, there's a good chance that your motivation will burn out and you'll lose the commitment to succeed. In a study of outpatients who were entering an alcohol-treatment program, researchers from the University of Rochester discovered that those who scored high on measures of internalized motivation were more likely to be active participants and to have the best attendance records throughout the treatment. In another study, researchers found that people who enrolled in a six-month weight-loss program because they were personally motivated to do so attended the program more regularly, lost more weight during the regimen, and maintained greater weight loss after two years.

There doesn't have to be a conflict between internal and external rewards. Some of the early research suggested that there was an inherent conflict—that there had to be an either-or choice—between internal motivation and external rewards; the theory was that external rewards would somehow extinguish internal motivation. But later research has suggested that this does not have to be the case, that internal and external rewards can actually fuel each other in some instances, especially if the external rewards are self-chosen.

Internal rewards can exert a strong emotional charge that can make you want to keep striving for your goals. But sometimes you may need a little outside assistance to help you stick with the process long enough or to reach a point where you can reap these benefits. Of course, bribing yourself with external gifts and incentives will only work for so long; if you don't find a way to enjoy the journey to change, you're unlikely to make it to your destination. But if you use the two forms of rewards compatibly, you can boost your motivation over the long run.

How to Start Your Own Incentives Program

While you're working hard to reach a goal, you should reward yourself for the progress you make and for your effort. It's all about positive reinforcement—rewarding positive behavior to promote more of the same. Instead of offering yourself a huge payoff at the end of the line, rewards are more helpful if they're tied to smaller measures of progress. That way, they'll encourage more of the behavior that immediately preceded the reward. Here are five ways to use incentives effectively:

1. Give yourself verbal pats on the back. This can be done when you reach small milestones by saying to yourself something like "Way to go!" as well as when you sidestep trouble. When you avoid a setback—whether it's giving in to the temptations of a buffet at a party or losing your cool during a stressful performance review at work—take some deep breaths and calmly praise yourself for maintaining control. These private kudos will reinforce the positive behavior you've just exhibited.

2. Offer yourself small treats. The idea isn't to spoil yourself but to reward yourself modestly for making strides toward your goal. If your aim is to train for a 10K race, you might reward yourself with a sports massage when you can comfortably jog three miles (the halfway point). If you're looking for a new job, you might treat yourself to a manicure after you've sent out 20 résumés. Also, make a wish list of things you would most appreciate in times of depletion or distress and use it to give yourself bonuses when you need them most. This will give you something to look forward to when you feel on the verge of giving up.

3. Make a deal with yourself. When you really don't feel like doing whatever task lies before you but you know you should, it's okay to resort to bargaining with yourself. Force yourself to plunge into the task at hand but give yourself permission to quit if doing it feels terrible after a reasonable time period. You might tell yourself that you can stop running after 10 or 15 minutes if it feels terrible—or that you can quit working on that dreaded report after an hour if you're not making any progress. The odds are, you'll stick with it after becoming invested in what you're doing.

4. Give yourself permission to hold on to the trophy. It doesn't have to be a real trophy or prize, but it should be some tangible acknowledgment (even a symbolic one will do) of what you've done—perhaps a certificate of excellence from a course that you took or a photograph of you crossing the finish line in a race. Research has found that being allowed to keep an end product of her efforts can enhance a person's performance on a task, spurring her to work longer on a chosen activity and boosting her senses of self-determination and competence afterward.

5. Write a contract with yourself. Contracts are powerful tools for promoting certain behaviors, and you can use this principle with yourself. Make an agreement with yourself in writing that for every week of consistent workouts, for every 10 résumés you send out, or for every afternoon that you volunteer in the community—or whatever action your goal entails—you'll place $10 in a spending account. (Alternatively, you could place two hours in a leisure-time account.) Then, when you need positive reinforcement to continue with your plan, you can withdraw from the account and reward yourself—by buying yourself a book (or another modest item) you've been wanting or by giving yourself some extra private time to spend as you please.

Learning to Appreciate Your Progress

Focusing on your progress as you pursue your goal helps you sustain motivation in several ways. For one thing, you can earn a sense of satisfaction over the good work you're doing every step of the way; you don't need to wait until you've attained your goal to gain gratification. And why should you? Why postpone happiness until after you've gotten that brilliant new career, slimmed down to your ideal weight, or completely revamped your lifestyle? The truth is, you could actually enjoy the journey and appreciate the small milestones along the way, which will make the trip to your ultimate goal that much easier and more pleasant. Most important, letting yourself feel satisfaction along the way can increase your capacity for happiness in your life.

In fact, it's a good idea to shift your focus slightly. Rather than view any challenge as an effort to get to and across a finish line, it's better and healthier to pay attention to your progress and all the experiences that come with it along the way. Think of achieving your goal more as the culmination of the natural unfolding of progress and less as the be-all-and-end-all result. This way, you'll be more likely to feel motivated throughout the pursuit and less likely to be discouraged by minor setbacks or to feel disappointed by the result if it doesn't happen exactly the way you envisioned it. Besides, there's an inherent satisfaction that comes with the realization that you're on a constructive track to self-improvement, that you are spending your time and energy in a worthwhile manner, which will boost your enthusiasm for investing more of your precious resources in pursuit of that goal. Although having a strong sense of purpose is essential in being motivated to take on a challenge, it's recognition of the progress you're making that is likely to sustain your motivation along the way because it protects you from burnout.

Tracking your progress also turns the pursuit of a goal into a learning experience by revealing which strategies seem to be working for you and which ones don't. Not only can you create various forms of feedback that will tell you how you're doing and what you might do differently, but you can use these to boost your confidence (especially if the feedback is positive) and your sense of being able to control the outcome. These benefits are likely to have a motivating effect because you'll see just how close you're coming to attaining your goals. And as you see the gap narrowing between where you are and where you want to be in terms of attaining your goals, you'll be inspired to work that much harder and smarter. Here are six ways to highlight your progress and bring it into sharper focus:

Keep a diary. Make a record of specific steps you take in pursuing your goal, how you felt while making them, what stumbling blocks you encountered (if any), and how you dealt with them. This is called self-monitoring, and besides making you accountable for your actions, it can help you see the consequences of what you do, especially in terms of what promotes progress and what doesn't.

In a study at the Center for Behavioral Medicine in Chicago of nearly 40 people who were trying to lose weight, researchers found that keeping a food diary not only helped them control their weight during high-risk holidays but even helped them shed unwanted pounds. Meanwhile, when researchers at the University of Texas School of Public Health in Houston conducted an analysis of studies examining techniques for changing certain health behaviors, they found that self-monitoring was especially helpful for people who were trying to quit smoking and drinking and for those who were attempting to improve their eating habits and slim down.

Become a trend tracker. Consider making a graph or chart to give you as much positive feedback as possible about your efforts. For example, if your goal is to make exercise a habit, you might keep a graph that shows the length and frequency of your workouts. This will automatically encourage you to keep a participatory trend going; plus, if you consider how much easier your workouts get over time, that's added incentive to keep up the good work. Likewise, if you want to find a new job, draw up a chart that illustrates how many résumés you send and how many phone calls you make each week in search of new opportunities; the more feelers you send out into the professional world, the more responses you're likely to get, which will keep you motivated to keep at it.

Focus on becoming more aware of your mind and body. Pay attention to psychological details such as a rising sense of confidence, feeling better about yourself, or an upswing in your mood, as well as physical improvements you feel. Once you've begun to make exercise a habit, you might notice that you're beginning to feel stronger throughout your body; as you gain more experience going on job interviews, you might realize that you're breathing easier or standing taller as you become more comfortable presenting yourself to strangers in a professional setting. Not only does focusing on your mind/body signals help you stay connected to what you're doing, it also helps you notice small improvements in how you're feeling as you pursue your goal.

Mark your milestones—even the little ones. Milestones are especially important when it comes to long-term goals such as losing a significant amount of weight, dramatically improving your health or creating an entirely new career for yourself, because the progress may be very gradual and the desired goal a relative speck on the horizon. By breaking up your goal into psychologically significant advances, it will help you experience your fair share of successes along the way, which will help keep you energized for the long haul.

The way to do this is to work backward from a long-term goal and delineate smaller stepping-stones that will help you get there—and to pause long enough to let yourself celebrate your arrival at each one. If your goal is to run a marathon, you might pay special attention to the satisfaction you feel when you can feel comfortable running 6.5 miles (one-quarter of the distance), 13 miles (the halfway point), and 19.5 miles (three-quarters of the distance); this way, you'll feel proud of yourself along the way and motivated to continue your training. Just be sure to stop and savor the sweet taste of satisfaction before moving forward again. (You'll learn more about how to set short-term versus long-term goals in Chapter 6.) In other words, give yourself credit for what you've already done. Remember: Even small improvements count, and they certainly add up to a higher quality of life.

Ask others for input. You don't want other people to start policing your actions, but it can be helpful to get feedback occasionally on what you've been doing. After all, other people have a more objective, less biased perspective on how well you're doing as you strive for a goal. When you do ask trusted friends, family members or colleagues for input, ask them to be very specific about what they see. Having a colleague tell you "Your presentation was really great" isn't nearly as helpful as "I thought your ideas about how to improve the company's market share were really creative. But I think you should use more visual aids in your talks." This way, you'll get a precise idea about what you should work to improve.

Increase the fun factor. Are you having fun yet? As you pursue your goal, it's important to ask yourself periodically whether you're enjoying what you're doing and to consider how you might make the experience even more pleasant. If your training regimen is starting to feel ho-hum, you might inject a little variety by trying some new activities. If you're getting sick and tired of sending out résumé after résumé, why not attend a networking event and schmooze a little to broaden your contact list? Not only is keeping your pursuits fun important for sustaining motivation, it's an essential aspect of taking good care of yourself psychologically and emotionally.

Discovering the Power of Flow

All of the elements that are essential to internal motivation—choice, purpose, mastery and progress—are intricately intertwined. Each one exerts a strong, synergistic influence on the others. And while each element, by itself, can help bolster your motivation, together they are a most powerful reinforcement. When they work well in concert, like a finely tuned orchestra, you can achieve a sense of inner harmony and a psychological state called "flow," an optimal frame of mind in which you are totally absorbed in what you are doing.

Research has found that people who are highly motivated, especially those who are internally motivated, tend to experience flow more often. A recent study from the University of Ottawa found that master's-level swimmers who were internally motivated to succeed or participate and who felt autonomous and competent were more likely to experience flow during a swim practice than those who were unmotivated.

When people experience a state of flow, they typically feel strong, alert, in effortless control, and at the peak of their abilities, according to research by the father of flow, Mihaly Csikszentmihalyi, Ph.D., a professor of psychology at the University of Chicago. Basically, achieving a state of flow can become its own reward, not to mention a powerful incentive to continue doing whatever it was that brought you to that optimal experience. People can achieve this heightened state of performance and enjoyment through all sorts of different activities—playing sports, working at their jobs, dancing, playing music, engaging in hobbies, socializing, even reading with their children. And the language people use to describe how they feel when they're involved in activities that are going especially well is remarkably similar. (Interestingly enough, a study of 78 adults found that the great majority of flow experiences were reported when people were working, not when they were pursuing leisure activities.)

The good news is, this state doesn't just happen by chance. There are actually steps you can take to create a climate that's conducive to flow. And it's worth the effort because once you achieve flow, you'll be in a state where you have a surplus of motivation for the goals you've set your sights on—and you'll be willing to expend an enormous amount of energy just to be able to feel that sensation again.

Knowing You're in the Flow

According to research by Csikszentmihalyi, the phenomenon of flow has the following fundamental elements: There's an equal balance between a person's capabilities or skills and the challenges that are involved in a task or situation. Because a person's attention and skills are completely absorbed in the activity, action and awareness become so thoroughly blended that she is no longer aware of herself as separate from what she is doing. The situation's goals are well defined and feedback is automatic. During the activity, a person's concentration is completely focused on the task at hand. She has a feeling of control—or she's not worried about losing control—over herself and the environment. There is a loss of consciousness of the self that takes place; a person's self-concept and self-scrutiny, which are a part of her normal, everyday life, simply slide outside of her awareness. There is a sense that time has been suspended, as if in a dream. And, finally, the experience itself is so intrinsically enjoyable that it becomes an end in itself.

Obviously, you can't control whether all of these elements will occur. But you can set yourself up for the possibility that flow will happen by creating flow-friendly conditions. One of the keys to doing this is to set clear goals that fairly match your capabilities or skills against challenges and to choose activities that are bounded by stable rules (rather than chaos). Then, it's up to you to cultivate the ability to concentrate by focusing all of your attention and efforts on the task at hand and by staying alert to feedback from the environment.

You'll also need to be willing to allow a sense of self-consciousness to melt away—a challenge for any woman, but particularly for one who has struggled with her weight. If possible, try to forget about how you look and how you're doing; simply focus intently on what you're doing. Among the hidden benefits to forgetting who you are as you participate in a challenging activity is that it will probably end up strengthening your self-concept. Because you are challenged to do your best and to give your all in a flow experience, afterward, when you have a chance to reflect upon what has occurred, the self that you see will be enhanced by your refined skills and newest accomplishment.

Once you begin to let these elements happen, the rest will be easier to realize as the flow experience assumes a life of its own. At that point, motivation will cease to be an issue because you'll be so fully invested in what you are doing. Best of all, this will help you learn to enjoy life in the moment and maintain an overall sense of purpose for your life, one that will propel you forward to a richer, more satisfying existence.

ASSIGNMENT By this point, you should be fairly clear about what gives your life a sense of meaning or purpose. (If you need a refresher on this, take another look at your notes from Chapter 2.) Now make a list of goals that would add new meaning to your life and why they are important to you. Next, consider how you intend to act on them. What aspects of the process of pursuing those goals do you think will be valuable, interesting or enjoyable by themselves? How can you naturally tap into that intrinsic source of motivation along the way? Make a list of ways you can do that right here—and refer to it as needed in the future.

CHAPTER FIVE

Turn Off the Autopilot

When you stop and think about it, we're all creatures of habit. Despite the fact that I'm constantly on the run and forever traveling, I always bring my habits along with me wherever I go. Like most people, I'm barely aware of the things I routinely do. I fiddle nervously with my hair, a harmless habit and one that's somehow comforting for me. I also tap my toe when I'm impatient, hum when I'm happy, and doodle on paper while I'm thinking.

I have my share of bad habits, too, but nothing compares to the insidious habit of emotional binge eating. The root of the problem lies somewhere in my childhood, when eating became something more than just sustenance. Back then and to this day, things like creamy egg and mayonnaise sandwiches, country ham, warm buttery toast, and any variety of cheese are deeply comforting to me. As a young girl these foods made me feel secure and loved. After my parents' divorce I found that eating calmed my nerves and filled the emotional void left in our broken home.

As a teenager my eating habits were already out of control. I'd eat with my friends to celebrate and eat in private to compensate for my shortcomings. The pattern of my youth followed me right into my adult life, where the cycle of binge eating and starving became a real problem. I look back now with informed perspective and realize I was out of control—and completely unaware of it.

I couldn't agree more with the premise of this chapter, "Turn Off the Autopilot," because it addresses that dreadful feeling you get when your life is in a tailspin and you feel incapable of doing much about it. That's what happened to Weight Watchers leader Jenn Thomas. She is proof that even in free fall you can still grab the wheel of change and veer off to a new and better life.

It's interesting that Jenn's mother's success on Weight Watchers gave her hope about her own weight problem. I feel strongly that parents can help give their children a healthier and happier life by setting a good example. I use the knowledge and skills that I use daily to control my weight to teach and nurture my daughters, who, thankfully, are not comfort eaters. At the end of last summer's vacation, just before returning to school, Beatrice and Eugenie and I began talking about their need to be more aware of nutrition. After a summer of too many sodas, cookies and pizza, they were more than eager to join me in a healthy and balanced diet. Now the girls know they can join me in following the program whenever they like, and when they do we help keep each other on track.

But Jenn had to make the change herself, and she acknowledges that it took a string of little steps to get motivated and to have a plan of action for losing weight. None of us became overweight overnight and it's important to be realistic about the fact that weight doesn't come off fast. In fact, fast weight loss can have terrible health risks, which is reason enough to gear yourself up for what we like to call the "journey" toward your healthy weight. It's more than a diet, and you'll discover parts of yourself along your journey that'll change you on the inside as well as the outside as you reach your goal.

Jenn's success proves the power of setting and achieving small goals. She also can attest to the power of positive attitude, which we need to foster in ourselves. When we are living on autopilot we let the opinions of others influence our self-worth. What a liberating feeling it is when we learn to take steps that affect our mood and direction in life. When we learn to believe in ourselves we are more willing to take challenges, and that is the start of self-discovery.

Listen to what Jenn has to say about exercise, too, because she gradually added physical activity to her life, which not only helped her sustain progress in shedding pounds but enabled her to see the positive psychological benefits that came from moving her body. She told me that she does not go to a gym and that her fitness regimen of simple stretches, walking and running are things she can do right at home. I'm the same way, because I hate having to go out and put on gym outfits and then wash my hair again after working out. I much prefer the time I spend on the stationary bike in the comfort and privacy of my home or the freedom of doing some simple exercises in a hotel room while traveling. All it takes is getting your heart going for 20 minutes every day and you'll begin to see the benefits.

Profile: JENN THOMAS
Becoming Mindful of My Actions

As if the teenage years weren't hard enough, adding unwanted inches and pounds during this emotionally tumultuous time can make a girl feel downright shaky about herself. If anyone knows this it's Jenn Thomas, now 28, a math and science teacher in New York, who used food as a crutch for her insecurities during adolescence. "I was a closet eater so no one would see me," she confesses. "I wouldn't eat in front of anyone. It was sporadic but when I felt low, I'd try to separate myself and I'd eat foods I liked, Devil Dogs, Twinkies, Doritos, and that kind of thing." Not surprisingly, these secretive indulgences added up to weight gain.

When her mother joined Weight Watchers, Jenn decided to try to lose weight, too. "I just sat in the meetings with her, and that's how it began," recalls Jenn, who is 5 feet 10 inches and does jazz and tap dancing as a hobby. "It wasn't easy. It took me a year to lose 30 pounds, and three different times I gained 20 of it back. The reason I gained is I never offered myself change and flexibility. And I really struggled with motivation. I didn't think I could do it. I kept setting myself up for failure because failure felt more comfortable to me. I had these little rules—if no one was there, I could eat whatever I wanted. It didn't count if I ate in the train station on my way to or from school. My thought processes were a little weak."

Finally, Jenn decided to take control of her behavior by reclaiming control of her mind-set. Instead of just reaching for food on a whim, she became more mindful of her eating habits—by chewing her food slowly and putting her fork down between bites. By choosing to graze healthfully all day long because that's what works for her. By stopping when she feels good instead of continuing to eat until she feels full or bloated. And by always sitting down and eating from a plate, instead of out of the refrigerator. "When I was overweight, I used to eat on an unconscious level; I didn't really enjoy food or taste it," Jenn admits. "Now I'm more mindful of what I'm doing. I'm really chewing it and enjoying the flavor when I eat, and that helps me enjoy it more."

She even started writing down ahead of time what she planned to eat. "I would set goals for the day," she recalls. "I would try to drink more water or aim to eat more vegetables on a particular day. I started exercising in little ways, by going walking with a friend or doing exercises while watching TV. I wouldn't overwhelm myself with a lot of goals. I'd set just one for the day, and if I made it, I'd have a good day. Thirty pounds may not sound like a lot to people, but it was what my body was used to so it was hard for me to lose." Jenn got in the habit of setting small goals—losing five-pound increments, for example—and rewarding herself with a new haircut, a manicure, a massage, a special dance class, or some other form of self-pampering when she reached a goal.

Jenn also began setting herself up for good days by giving herself pep talks and adopting what she calls "thin attitudes." She kept a picture of her thin self around for constant inspiration and learned to stop berating herself for what she perceived as her physical flaws. Instead, she began writing herself positive messages on Post-its, things like "Keep up with your success" or "Remember your goals and dreams. You can achieve them," and she'd leave them all over her apartment or stick them in her day planner. "I started looking in the mirror and saying I can do this, and You deserve to lose the weight," she recalls. "When I started losing weight, I started telling myself, You do look good; you can look better. Before I'd eat something, I'd ask myself, Do you really want this? or Where will this dessert really go? Probably to my hips, where I didn't want it. Even today, when I eat something I think I shouldn't have, as I'm eating it, I think about what time I'm going to start eating healthfully again. Or I think about what I'm going to eat tomorrow. I basically try to refocus my thoughts. To this day, the minute my pants start fitting differently I look at where I went wrong and try to refocus."

This present-mindedness, this focus on living consciously, may have been sparked by her desire to slim down, but it has carried over into other areas of Jenn's life as well. "It's also made me more mindful in teaching, my dancing, and my friendships," she says. "It makes me think about what's happening in these areas and what I'm doing, what the outcome might be. I feel more confident now; my positive self-image has been brought out. And I'm really there in the moment. I don't think I used to be mindful of where I was and what I was doing. Losing the weight really made me start to stand up for myself and say what was on my mind. I was able to free my emotions, which had been held inside."

Ever since she lost weight, Jenn hasn't been afraid to go out on a limb and take chances. Among her crowning achievements: "It gave me the self-confidence to walk up to my future husband in the park and say, 'Hi. How are you?'" she recalls. After a long courtship, the couple married in the summer of 2000.

Indeed, the payoff for losing weight proved to be much greater than Jenn had originally hoped. "I started operating more quickly; I wasn't as sluggish," she explains. "And I stopped procrastinating as much. It made me socialize with friends more. I had been more of a follower, and Weight Watchers made me say 'I am special. I can be a leader.'" Indeed, she credits becoming a Weight Watchers leader with helping her to stay strong. "As much as I empower the people in my meetings, they motivate me," Jenn explains. "They're very supportive and they look up to me and they want me to teach them as much as possible. That makes me feel like I need to prove myself to myself and to them.

"Living mindfully is going to guarantee me that I'll lead a thinner life and not go back to where I was 10 years ago," she says. "It helps me stay aware of my goals and dreams, and it makes me realize I need to take slow action steps instead of going for instant gratification. I've also learned to be happy with the small rewards, which will eventually lead to the big goals—and that's true of any area of my life."

IT'S TIME TO CONFESS: How many times have you made New Year's resolutions that you never followed through on? If you're like most people, it's probably happened too many times for you to count. And there's a reason for this; actually, there are a few. For one thing, we've become such a goal-oriented society that many people have fallen into the habit of setting goals without giving any real thought to what's involved in actually striving for them. Maybe they decide they're inspired to lose weight after seeing an old friend who did it but they're not clear about why *they* want to tackle this challenge. Or maybe they realize they want to get a promotion at work without having any concrete sense of how to go about earning one. Or maybe they vow to lead a healthier lifestyle but they fail to pay attention to exactly what that entails on a daily basis. When you think about it, it's hardly surprising that people who fall into these patterns often abandon their goals within a short time.

How could it be any other way? After all, one of the keys to getting what you want in life is to make mindful choices in both the short term and the long term. So many people go through life, either vaguely aware of their desires or focused exclusively on the immediate situation or on instant gratification, and as a result, they don't really think about what they're doing. Consequently, they aren't likely to improve their lives substantially because they aren't in tune with what they really want—or with whether they're helping or hindering their ability to achieve it. They are moving through life on automatic pilot or cruise control instead of actively driving the car. As Ellen Langer, Ph.D., a professor of psychology at Harvard University, notes, the roots of mindlessness are deeply embedded, and in the course of daily living, people tend to realize they are operating on this level only when an acute problem occurs. But even if it doesn't lead to a crisis, staying on automatic pilot can slowly but surely chip away at the quality of your life or stunt your potential for personal growth.

So how do you get back behind the wheel? It starts with viewing yourself as an agent of change, as commander of your own destiny. Coming up with a mission can help turn off the automatic pilot because you're no longer just coasting aimlessly. Your self-chosen mission gives you direction in your life, and that can help you emerge from a mental fog. The next challenge is to make sure that your actions will take you there.

To ensure that this happens, you'll need to cultivate self-awareness, for starters, but also self-control, proactivity and mindfulness. Simply put, self-awareness means that you are conscious of your own actions and you have an understanding of how you behave and react. Self-control is essentially a matter of being able to regulate your own behavior. Being proactive means taking action that's in line with your goals, values and your guiding sense of purpose in life, rather than simply reacting to life's circumstances. And mindfulness involves focusing your attention on what you are doing and experiencing from one moment to the next. Developing these qualities will help you become more cognizant of the little things you do on a daily basis, and help you become the person that you want to be.

The Secrets to Becoming Mindful

Of course, it's not enough to set goals constructively, launch your plan of action and then simply hope for the best. You'll need to keep tabs on all the little things you do on a daily basis that could promote or undermine your efforts. One of the best ways to do this is to cultivate mindfulness. Mindfulness is a concept that refers to the practice of becoming fully attentive to what you are experiencing in the present moment. You don't let your mind wander to the past or the future; you simply focus your full awareness on the thoughts and experiences that are occurring right now. It also involves expanding your definition of yourself—beyond the fixed roles you may occupy—and tapping into skills and strengths you may have overlooked. As Vietnamese Zen master Thich Nhat Hanh once wrote: "Mindfulness is the miracle by which we can call back in a flash our dispersed mind and restore it to wholeness so that we can live each minute of life."

Not only can being mindful help you live each day more fully, but it can even help you improve your health. Research has found that mindfulness meditation—combining the practice of mindfulness with a focus on your breathing or on the act of walking—can relieve pain, reduce stress, and improve specific health conditions. A study conducted at the Center for Mindfulness in Medicine at the University of Massachusetts in Worcester found that using mindfulness meditation to reduce stress helped patients with psoriasis heal faster when they were undergoing phototherapy. Other studies have found that mindfulness meditation can improve anxiety and panic disorders. And a recent study from Connecticut discovered that the technique helped people who were participating in a stress-reduction program at a community health center change their attitudes, beliefs, habits and behaviors; in addition to improving physical and psychological symptoms that were related to stress, these people experienced an upswing in their self-esteem.

Changing Bad Habits

When it comes to changing your ways and striving for your goals in life, sometimes you can be your own worst enemy. But this isn't about teaching you how to remember to put the cap back on the toothpaste (an annoying habit, but relatively benign in the grand scheme of things). It's better to expend your time and energy trying to free yourself from the patterns of behavior that are truly self-sabotaging. That's because bad habits—such as overeating, being sedentary, smoking, procrastinating, being disorganized, and so on—really stem from a state of *mindlessness*. These habits can make you inefficient or, worse, impair your progress toward your goals; resorting to them is rather like keeping one foot on the brake and the other on the accelerator as you're driving. We're all creatures of habit, and while bad habits may be hard to break, they're not impossible.

One of the first essential elements of changing self-limiting habits is to develop self-awareness, to begin to understand when you usually engage in the behavior and what purpose it serves for you. The best way to track habits is to keep a journal, in which you note every time you engage in the behavior and what the external and internal (or emotional) circumstances were. Doing this will help you draw connections between when you do it and why you do it.

Once you have this information, you can use mindfulness and substitution strategies to redirect your behavior. (Even becoming mindful of your actions can help you break small annoying habits. If you adopt a pattern of forcing yourself to pause for a moment after brushing your teeth, for example, you can make yourself remember to replace the cap on the toothpaste.) When you catch yourself falling into an old pattern, stop yourself in your tracks, take a deep breath and focus on what you are doing. Then ask yourself: Do I

continued on next page

really want to do this? Will my actions help or hinder my goals? What would I be better off doing instead?

These three simple questions can help you avert all kinds of self-impairing behavior, from overeating and being sedentary to procrastinating or worrying needlessly. For example, if you tend to spend too much time noshing at cocktail parties and you want to lose weight, you might stop yourself before reaching for a plate and ask yourself: Am I really hungry? Will filling up on fat-laden hors d'oeuvres help or hinder my weight-loss goals? Would I be better off having a glass of seltzer and socializing instead? Or, if you often put off working on reports until the eleventh hour but you want to do an especially good job on a project that's due next week, you might ask yourself now: Do I really want to wait until the last minute to write this? Will procrastinating help or hinder my desire to do a first-rate job? Wouldn't I be better off getting started now so that I'll have plenty of time to deal with glitches that come up and to polish the final product?

By presenting the situation to yourself in such clear terms, the incentive to try behaving another way will likely become compelling. After all, it's hard to change your behavior until you've convinced yourself that it's in your best interest to do so. This technique can help you instantly envision the benefits of trying another way.

If you then talk yourself through the process of doing things differently step by step, you'll help yourself maintain control over the situation rather than reverting to unhealthy patterns. And if you regularly use this exercise to help you short-circuit self-destructive habits and replace them with more constructive ones, these helpful forms of behavior will gradually become second nature to you. You'll use them without having to think about it, and then you'll feel like you're driving yourself toward your goals with one foot squarely on the accelerator, which is as it should be.

With mindfulness, the key is to be open and receptive to what you are experiencing. To do that, you'll need to take off your blinders or distorting or rose-colored lenses and try to see situations objectively. You'll need to consciously try to slow down and pay attention to nuances—particularly in how you feel and in what's happening around you—throughout the day. You'll need to reclaim enough control over the pace of your life that you'll be able to see your actions clearly and be able to evaluate, often in a split second, whether you are inclined to do what's really in your best interest. Here are eight simple ways to cultivate mindfulness:

1. Remind yourself that you're constantly making choices. Take responsibility for the myriad decisions you make on a daily basis. When you help yourself to a second serving of birthday cake, decide not to throw your hat in the ring for a coveted promotion at work, or you forgo your morning jog on a chilly morning, remind yourself, I am making this choice and this is my choice and my choice alone to make. In the end, each and every action you take or choose not to take is up to you.

2. Write down the important stuff. It may sound too mundane to be helpful when you're pursuing lofty ambitions, but writing it down is like making a contract with yourself. It serves as a tangible reminder of what you should be doing when you become distracted and can help you stay in touch with what you're intentionally trying to do. Finally, it frees your mind from the shackles of having to remember what you should be doing. Trying hard not to forget something is an energy drainer; redirct that energy to achieving the goals you've set your sights on.

3. Build in a pause. Stop what you are doing, take a deep breath and think about what you *really* want to do in a particular situation before making a decision. Ask yourself: Do I really want to do what I'm naturally inclined to do? Will this serve my goals well in the short term and the long term? What might happen if I did something else, even the opposite? In these hectic times, it's all too easy to get swept up in the moment and swing into action. But you can actually choose to stop and take the time you need to decide how you'd like to respond or act in a given situation. Whether it takes a few seconds, minutes or days, it's time well spent.

4. Focus on the present. So many people spend the majority of their lives dwelling on the past, the regrets they have, what might have been; or looking to the future, fantasizing about what could happen or worrying about what might be. If you're so focused on alternate time frames, you won't be experiencing what's happening here and now as fully as you could. The reality: There are lots of yesterdays and plenty of tomorrows but only one today.

The idea isn't to live your life in such a moment-to-moment fashion that you lose sight of your guiding values or mission. What you want to do is to focus on what you can do *right now* that's in sync with those elements. After all, the present is where your life is happening now.

5. Learn how to listen. Most of us spend too much time talking and too little time really listening to what's being said to us or around us. But if you actually make the effort to listen actively, you can absorb all kinds of useful information. Maybe someone else's bad-luck love story will turn out to be a cautionary tale for you and alert you to subtle signs of trouble in your own relationship. Or maybe a colleague's gripes about the company will give you ideas about how to boost employee morale and productivity—ideas you could then share with your boss.

There are several ways to hone your listening skills: You can conjure up a visual image of what's being said; you can try to zero in on the essential facts or messages and weed out the fluff; or you can use reflective techniques such as repeating what someone has just told you, using your own words. Whichever method you choose to use, you'll be treating yourself to a richer experience.

6. Become more grounded in everyday life. Focus your attention on what's going on around you and don't let your mind wander. You could do this formally by learning to meditate and practicing for, say, 15 or 20 minutes every day. Or you can do this in all sorts of little ways. When you wake up in the morning, you might start the day by paying attention to the rhythm and depth of your breathing and how the air feels as it enters your body, rather than immediately thinking about what's on today's agenda. Instead of rushing off to work with your head in a spin, make an effort to notice and appreciate something new in your surroundings, whether it's blossoms on a tree, the pattern of clouds in the sky or the scent of jasmine in the park. During the day, take mini breaks at your desk and pay attention to signs of tension in your body; perform some gentle stretches or relaxation exercises to ease the kinks. Stay connected to the subtle messages your body and mind send you as you go about the business of your life and try to build in restorative time as needed. By regularly putting these measures into practice, you're retraining your body and your mind to be more centered and invested in what's happening now.

7. *Isolate the elements.* When something goes poorly in one area of your life, don't let it color your whole world. Try to be mindful of the fact that experiencing a setback on your weight-loss plan or losing money in an investment plan or receiving a less than stellar performance review at work doesn't mean your whole life is in shambles—it means theres a single problem that should be addressed.

When you can begin to see obstacles or setbacks in this light, they become less overwhelming and easier to deal with. Try to identify or define the specific problem, think of many different possible solutions, evaluate the pros and cons of each, then choose the best option that's available. Don't always go with the logical choice, though. Use your intuition and feelings to guide you; after all, intuition is problem solving on an unconscious level—and it's often right if you listen to it.

8. *Stay in tune with your thoughts.* Shutting off the automatic pilot isn't just a matter of being in charge of your actions. It involves tapping into your thoughts and redirecting them when necessary. As the Stoic philosopher and Roman emperor Marcus Aurelius once noted, "Our life is what our thoughts make it."

Keep a log. When something upsetting happens—a colleague makes a rude remark to you, your car breaks down, or you had a fight with your spouse—write down a description of what occurred, the unedited thoughts that automatically came to mind, and how strongly you believe them to be true. Then, consider how you may have distorted the reality by engaging in all-or-nothing thinking, by jumping to conclusions, by blowing things out of proportion, by being unjustly critical of yourself or taking things too personally.

Now read over what you've written, objectively. Perhaps the colleague who was rude to you was simply in a bad mood and took it out on you. Maybe your car's breaking down was nothing more than a stroke of bad luck, rather than an example of how nothing seems to be going your way. Perhaps you and your partner fought because you're both under a lot of stress and you need to find healthy ways to decompress together. This sort of technique is at the core of cognitive-behavioral therapy, and it really can help you see and experience the world in a healthier, more enjoyable way.

As you make these subtle perceptual shifts from being on automatic pilot to becoming mindful, you'll naturally become more present- and process-oriented than future- or outcome-oriented. This is an important adjustment to make because it helps you focus on what you can do today to improve your life. It gives you a greater sense of control over your life, simply by making you aware of different options and opportunities. It helps you fine-tune your judgment and your approach to challenges, which can make you feel better about yourself. And, perhaps most important, becoming mindful lets you enjoy the fruits of your efforts now instead of asking you to defer satisfaction.

The Right Way to Set Goals

You might have a mission or a guiding vision of what you want for your life, but how does that translate into action? Dreams alone aren't going to help you improve your life. What you need is a clear description of your goals, because it's your goals—individually and collectively—that will deliver you to your chosen destination in life. Once you've mapped out your goals, you can begin to take giant steps toward making your dreams become reality. Research with athletes has found that simply setting concrete goals can help them improve their performance considerably.

When it comes to formulating your goals, it's important to couch them in positive, active terms. Instead of setting goals that begin with "Don't . . ." or "I will not . . ." consider the essence of your desired situation or outcome and structure your goal that way. But also think about what it will take on your part to make that goal happen and present it in a statement that begins with "I will . . ." or "I'm going to . . ." If you want to gain a promotion at work, for example, you might tell yourself, "I'm going to write a first-rate report that will catch my supervisor's attention." If you want to improve your health, you might say, "I'm going to quit smoking" or "I will start exercising for 30 minutes at least four times per week."

If you keep your goals specific, well defined, and upbeat, you'll be giving yourself clear direction and something precise to focus your efforts on. That's because, phrased in these terms, your goals become proactive or action-oriented, rather than passive or results-oriented. This places the burden on you to achieve the desired outcome, which is how it should be. If, up until now, you've expressed your dreams in terms of your desired results, don't be discouraged. You don't have to start from scratch; simply forget about the result for the moment and focus instead on what you can do to achieve that goal and what's within your control. It's a slight shift in perspective—from "Save money" to "I'm going to put aside $50 from every paycheck," from "Improve my marriage" to "I will set the alarm clock 30 minutes earlier so that we can start each day by having breakfast together."

Before reading any further, take some time to contemplate the outcome you desire, then reformulate your goals in terms of concrete steps you can take to achieve those results. A chart (see page 119) can be a useful tool.

The language behind your plan of action should tell you exactly what you need to do to get the results you crave—and your goals should be measurable. Ideally, the goals you set should be hard enough to be challenging but not so hard that they're virtually unattainable. There's no reason to strive for Mission Impossible when Mission Reasonable would be much more beneficial for your life and your sense of well-being. On the other hand, goals shouldn't be so easy that you don't have to work hard for them. Psychologists point out that it's a basic law of human nature that people make more of an effort and strive more diligently for things that are out of their reach—and they gain more satisfaction in the pursuit. When trying to figure out if a particular goal is realistic, take stock of the

	Desired Outcome	Actions That Will Take Me There
GOAL #1	Start my own business.	Come up with a business plan Secure financial backing Develop a marketing strategy
GOAL #2		
GOAL #3		
GOAL #4		
GOAL #5		

strengths and skills you already have that will help you reach your goal and note areas where you need to improve or to get help from others.

What you want to do is set short-term goals as stepping-stones to larger or more time-consuming ones. This will become the essence of your plan of action. If you want to start your own business, for example, your goals might be to come up with a business plan, to secure financial backing, to develop a marketing strategy, to choose a location for your headquarters and to hire the necessary personnel. If your mission is to lead a healthier lifestyle, your goals might be to identify your current eating habits, to have a physical exam (so that you can accurately assess your starting point), to take steps to improve your diet, to embark on a regular exercise program and to find ways to reduce or manage stress in your life. These goals proceed in a step-by-step fashion toward a particular mission or dream.

To make this process more manageable, it also may help to break your smaller or short-term goals into specific, concrete steps. Think about how you will organize your efforts by considering where you are now, where you want to end up, and what it will take for you to get there. If one of your goals is to secure financial backing for a new business, for example, you'll want to take note of how much money you already have dedicated to the project, how much more you'll need, and to whom you can turn for additional financing. Once you've identified those individuals or lending institutions, you can work on polishing your pitch and setting up appointments to meet with prospective lenders. Similarly, if one of your goals is to identify your current eating habits before starting a program of clean living, you might want to keep a food diary for a week or two, analyze the results (perhaps by comparing it to the USDA Food Guide Pyramid), then figure out what food groups you're over- or underconsuming and whether you have emotional triggers for eating.

Here is what your game plan might look like:

Action-Oriented Goals	Stepping-Stones
Secure financial backing for a new business.	1. Assess how much money I have dedicated to the project.
	2. Figure out how much more money I'll need.
	3. Identify possible lenders.
	4. Develop a persuasive pitch.
	5. Set up appointments to meet with prospective lenders.

Going through this analytical process will help you pinpoint what is involved at every step. When you approach goal setting in this way, it takes away some of the pressure and worry that typically revolve around striving to succeed; as long as you implement your plan of action, you can't possibly fail, because doing something to better yourself or improve your life is a measure of success by itself. At first, charting this course may seem time-consuming, but it will actually end up saving you time and effort in the long run; you'll know just what you need to do as you pursue your goals; you won't waste time spinning your wheels or having to come up with a new game plan every step of the way.

Building a Bridge to Your Dreams

If your ultimate goal is a daunting one, it may help to come up with a reverse plan: Imagine that you've already achieved the outcome you want, then work backward and figure out how you might have arrived there. First ask yourself: What did I do just before I reached my ultimate goal? What did I do before that step? And so on. One of the advantages to this technique is that it may help you see that there's more than one route to your chosen destination.

This is really about creating your own individual plan for changing your life; it's not about following someone else's blueprint or a cookie-cutter guide to effecting change. It's your unique touch that can work absolute magic. A study from the University of Texas at Austin found that individualizing strategies for lifestyle change was the single most important predictor of goal achievement among 95 people who were seeking to improve their lifestyles; in fact, personalizing the steps to change helped 42 percent of the participants achieve their goal after just 10 weeks.

Once you are clear about what your goals are, it will become much easier to make smart, guided decisions in nearly every aspect of your life. Of course, it's also wise to get a pulse on how striving for these goals will shape your day-to-day life. How long do you think it will take to accomplish your big-picture goal? What will that require in the way of time and effort on a daily or weekly basis? After you have an inkling of what's realistic, try to set a time frame for your goals—one that's reasonable and somewhat flexible, rather than one that's etched in stone. It may even help to create a timeline with milestones you'd like to reach along the way; this way, even if you fall behind time-wise, you can keep track of your progress, which will help sustain your motivation. When your goals are mapped out, start by doing one thing as soon as possible that will help you reach your first stepping-stone.

Along the way, don't forget to try to remind yourself now and then why you want to achieve a particular goal. As you saw in Chapter 5, being clear about why you want something gives your life a sense of purpose,

The Keys to Peak Performance

Have you ever wondered why you can finish the crossword puzzle more easily in the morning than after lunch? Or why your tennis serve seems more powerful in the late afternoon? These aren't flukes. On the contrary, the secret to doing anything better may be in the timing. This is because your body's circadian rhythms—those 24-hour sleep-wake cycles and body-chemistry fluctuations—play a role in determining how alert, coordinated or strong you are throughout the day.

This internal clock, which is regulated by the hypothalamus in the brain, can prime your mind and body for certain feats at specific times of day. It's possible to use your natural highs to your best advantage by dedicating your peak performance times to accomplishing the tasks you've set as priorities. But you can only do this if you're mindful and aware of when these hours of power occur and you've organized your day accordingly. Because we're all unique, these windows of maximal opportunity may be slightly earlier or later for different people so you'll need to see what works best for you. (If you're an early riser or a late-night person, for example, these ups and downs may occur a few hours earlier or later.) What follows is a guide to the best times and the worst times for your performance in various areas of life:

7 to 9 A.M. You've got built-in pain protection. Research has found that pain tolerance is highest in the early morning, probably because endorphins, the body's natural painkillers that are released by the brain, are produced in greater quantities during the night. As a result, this is a good time to schedule dentist appointments or other physically painful procedures.

8 to 11 A.M. Your mental muscle power peaks. As body temperature rises throughout the morning, so do mental acuity,

continued on next page

short-term memory, logical reasoning skills and decision-making abilities. This is a good window of opportunity for tackling the day's most mentally challenging tasks, whether it's making a presentation, holding a business meeting, solving problems, strategizing or cramming for an exam.

2 P.M. You are most likely to daydream. When researchers at the National Institute on Aging studied the frequency of daydreams over a 24-hour period, they found that this was prime time for daydreaming, probably thanks to shifts in hormone levels and body temperature. You can take advantage of this propensity for the mind to wander and harness those fanciful images for your most creative projects.

2 to 3 P.M. Your alertness will likely wane. Many people experience a midafternoon slump in energy, concentration and efficiency, and many attribute this to a postlunch change in blood sugar. But this temporary sleepiness has little to do with the midday meal and more to do with being biologically programmed for a short nap after lunch, according to Timothy Monk, Ph.D., director of the Human Chronobiology Program at the University of Pittsburgh School of Medicine. You may be able to counteract this effect somewhat with a brisk walk.

2:30 to 4 P.M. Your coordination will kick in. Not only does hand-eye coordination peak during this time, but so do manual dexterity and reaction time. Which means this is an excellent time for practicing a musical instrument, typing, building something or playing tennis or golf.

3 to 4 P.M. Your mental concentration will return. Alertness rises again and your mood will probably take an upward ascent as well, boosting your sense of well-being and vigor. What's more, long-term memory—the ability to retain material over the long haul—reaches its peak now, so this is a good time to get trained in a

continued on next page

new computer program or to study material you'll need to remember for a long time.

4 to 6 P.M. Your exercise session will be most rewarding. If you really want to get the most from your workouts, this may be the best time to exercise. Research has found that muscle strength and flexibility tend to peak in the late afternoon, and studies have found that aerobic and anaerobic (the energy source for bursts of speed) capacities tend to be 5 percent higher in the late afternoon than in the morning.

6 to 8 P.M. Your sensory appreciation peaks. One reason why eating a favorite food or savoring a glass of fine wine is especially enjoyable after a hard day's work may be because your senses of taste and smell are most acute in the early evening, according to Monk. Which suggests it may be wise to wait until this time to treat yourself to the gustatory pleasures you crave the most. That way, you'll reap the maximum enjoyment from the experience.

which is essential to sustaining motivation. Without this, when you hit an obstacle, you might begin to question whether your efforts are truly worthwhile. And the danger is that once your senses of determination and commitment start to falter, you're on a steep and slippery slope toward abandoning your cause. On the other hand, if you sustain the conviction that your goals are important to you and have a clear sense of *why* they matter, you'll be less likely to lose sight of them or to suffer a motivational crisis.

ASSIGNMENT Make a list of your best and worst habits and when you tend to use them. Do you see any patterns here? How could you accentuate the positive by putting your best habits to use in more areas of your life? Also, think about what you could do to change the worst ones or simply relinquish them and consciously replace them with more productive or constructive ones. Create a flow chart that illustrates how and when you can substitute better habits for the bad ones. If you look below the surface of the whole habit issue, you'll probably realize that being mindful is the key to finding a better way.

CHAPTER SIX

Environment and You

ver feel dissatisfied with yourself but you can't tell what's wrong? I for one am very grateful for the blessings bestowed on my family and me. Yet there are times when I feel emotionally depleted, overwhelmed by work or just lacking in focus.

Earlier in my life I'd either deny the fact that I was feeling this way, or I'd go to the other extreme, engaging in terrible self-deprecation or imposing on myself baseless guilt that only made matters worse.

We feel unhappiness on the inside, but the reason for it may be external factors that we don't even know are there. Let's call them environmental factors, and they can really clutter up the little bubble we call our personal lives. I recall the nagging (at times overwhelming) loneliness I began to feel shortly after my marriage. Within weeks of our wedding Prince Andrew returned to active duty in the Royal Navy, which kept us apart all but 40 days a year. I'd assumed a very busy and high-profile life, which occupied most of my time by day—a dazzling whirlwind life fit for a fairytale princess—and I was puzzled about why I felt so unhappy despite the honor and privilege I enjoyed. The truth was, I was too busy to stop and look at my private Sarah. I was so eager to please everyone else amid my overloaded schedule that there just wasn't time left to address my own emotional needs.

You would think that living in a palace, where the kitchen is two miles away from your apartment, would be the magical solution for someone battling with her weight. But I think years of living separated from the man you love could drive any woman to despair. My solution to lessen the distance between my emotional hunger and the kitchen was to store goodies in the cupboard, like a squirrel hiding her acorns. I felt so clever, but in fact it only made matters worse, because I was discovered and suffered the guilt of a closet eater.

In this chapter, Weight Watchers leader Sharon Riguzzi talks about how environmental factors can play a big part in our weight problem. I've had the pleasure of knowing Sharon since I started my work with Weight Watchers in 1996, and I can tell you it is hard to imagine this beautiful, buoyant and confident woman ever feeling sad or stuck in a rut. And yet this is exactly where she found herself despite the blessings of a loving husband and family.

We say that hindsight is 20/20, and that's good *if* we can learn from our past experience. When I look back at my life during my most turbulent years I can see how much my environment fed into my weaknesses. This is not to blame others for my problems or to appear ungrateful for the amazing good fortune that I've had all of my life. What I am saying, though, is that had I known then what I know now, I'd be far better prepared to take some control over my surroundings and keep them from undermining my confidence and ability to grow. There are areas of my past that I still deeply regret, and in my talks with Weight Watchers leaders I'm often asked about moving on while living with regret. I've had to come to terms with my past because a lot of my troubles arose from not taking into account the consequences of my actions. To return to the river analogy, if I had only taken the corners in a more rounded fashion and kept my eyes open, I probably would have avoided a lot of trouble for myself.

Sharon says that one of the keys to her success was giving her environment a makeover. She knew she needed to get her weight under control, and as a woman who had been to Weight Watchers earlier in life, she understood that she had to make lasting lifestyle changes in order to get her weight off and keep it off. What I admire so much about Sharon is that she enlisted the support of others who cared enough to see her succeed, including her mother-in-law, whom she credits as being the best Italian cook ever.

I'll go one step further to say that honesty with yourself and others about your challenge is very important. We need to take the reins and control our destiny, but that does not mean that we need to do it alone. Moreover, it's not to say that others in our life can't benefit from the environmental changes we make.

Profile: SHARON RIGUZZI
Making My Life Support My Goals

We all know that old habits die hard, but Sharon Riguzzi is especially familiar with this unfortunate fact of life. What started as a mild case of baby fat turned into a bona fide weight problem when Sharon became a teenager and a college student, largely because she was eating her heart out. "I would eat for any emotion: stress, happiness, anger, depression," recalls Sharon, 48, a Weight Watchers leader in New York and a training manager for the eastern region. "I had joined Weight Watchers many different times since college. I would lose some weight and think I had this under control, then I'd stop coming. But I wouldn't really change anything. I'd diet then go back to my old habits and gain weight."

After marrying a man from an Italian family, whose mother was a fabulous cook and frequently prepared homemade ravioli and cannolis, Sharon gained more weight. "When I met my husband and I was introduced to all this wonderful food, it was like getting a great Christmas present," explains Sharon, whose family of origin was Irish. "I felt like I had to make up for all those years of not eating this food. I was enjoying myself to death."

Finally, in 1978, Sharon decided she wanted to make a concerted effort to slim down. "I decided to do this for me—not to look good in a bathing suit or to get a boyfriend, but for me," she recalls. The motivating factor: One day the paperboy was making the rounds, asking for donations, and Sharon's husband answered the door. The boy asked if his mother was home. "We all laughed," Sharon recalls, "because we always knew the paperboy wasn't all there. But then I went into the bathroom and cried. I didn't want to look like I was my husband's mother. He's older than I am and I knew it was the weight that was making me look older." She decided it was time to head back to Weight Watchers. But because Sharon was concerned about alienating her mother-in-law if she stopped eating the woman's fine cooking, Sharon invited

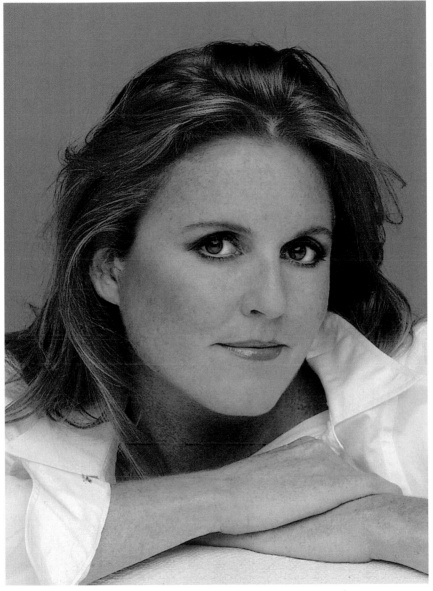

The photographer said, "Make love to the camera," but I was thinking something much different in this shot. Actually, I'm far more comfortable these days having my photo taken. I think my improved confidence and inner peace show through.

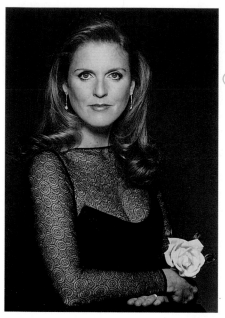

I say take a positive step forward after your thirty-ninth year and prove to the world that life begins at forty.

It was a wonderful day when I got my private pilot's license. My handsome husband, also a pilot, was very proud of what I'd accomplished.

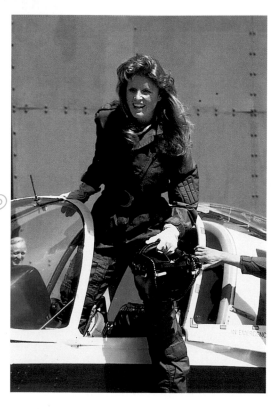

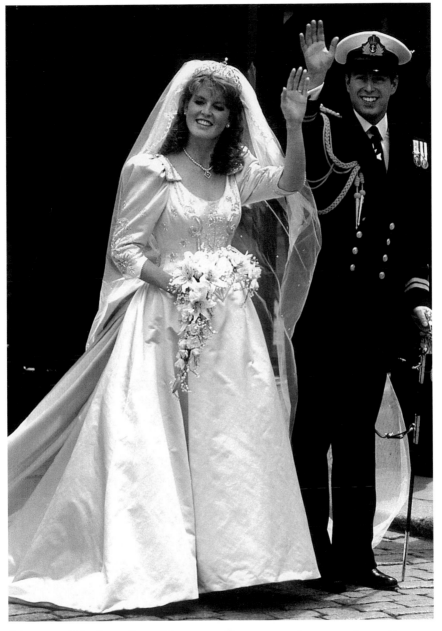

It's very difficult to live with regret. I've come a long way in putting my past mistakes into proper perspective, but deep in my heart I'll always wish that circumstances had not pulled our marriage apart. We were in the purest sense the happiest couple alive.

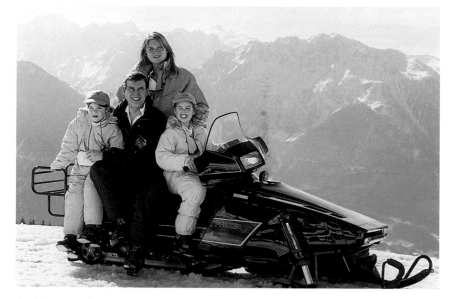

In Verbier, Switzerland, 1998, after our divorce. Divorce was devastating for me but thank heavens for the depth of our love and friendship that keeps us unified as a family.

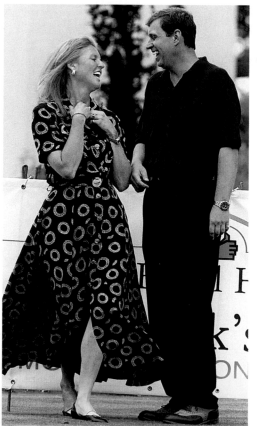

I have no better friend in the world than Andrew. Together we love being parents, and we keep our sense of humor all the time by looking at life with a positive smile. We still attend some of our favorite charity events together, this one recently at the Wentworth Golf Club near London for the Motor Neuron Disease Association Golf Tournament.

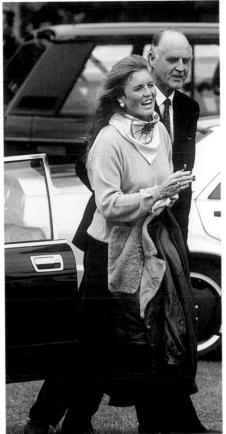

My wonderful father was very strict but unconditionally loving. Thank goodness I did not inherit his bushy eyebrows! Actually, when I look at this I look quite a lot like my mother, which thrills me.

My most special and beautiful mother, how I miss her so much! This was taken shortly before she died and it reminds me how Mum could bring light to a dark room. She always supported me through everything, including this art exhibit for my foundation Children in Crisis.

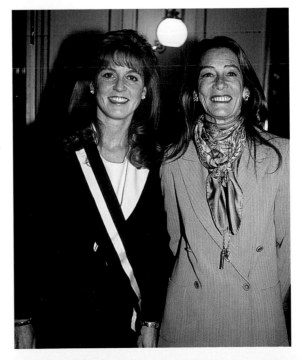

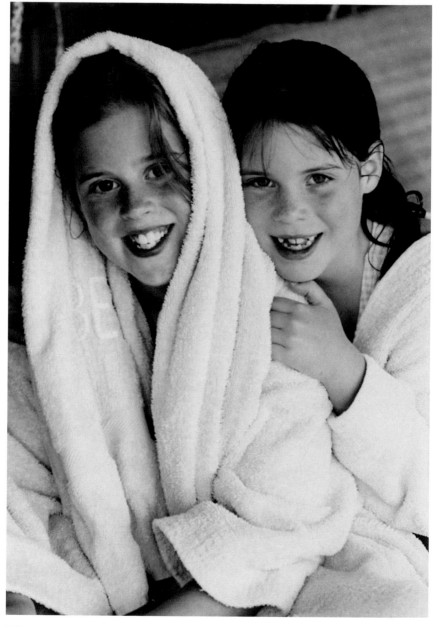

My girls, Beatrice and Eugenie, are shining satellites and like comets spraying pixie dust as they pass. They bring me enormous joy and pride every single day.

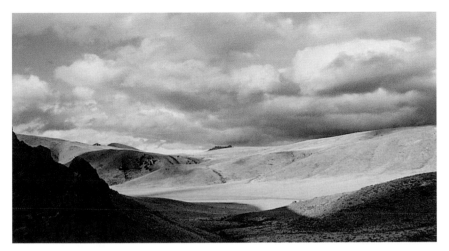

I took this photograph in the south of Argentina near Bariloche where the rocks on the horizon made me think of an ancient Greek city.

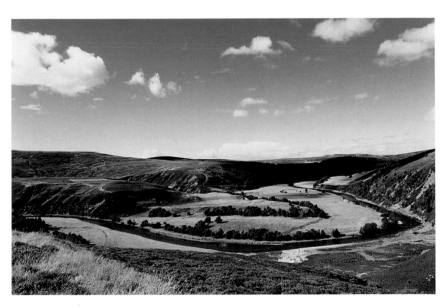

View from Drynachan Lodge in Scotland. I am The Countess of Inverness as well as The Duchess of York, and so I feel great affinity for Inverness. Being that I am half Scottish through my father, I feel a spiritual connection to this timeless and magnificently beautiful place.

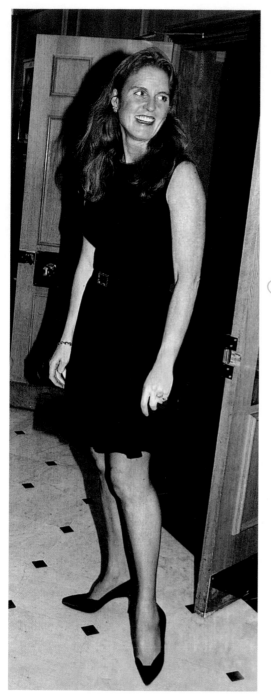

Normally I think I look big in photographs, but after practicing the Weight Watchers Tools for Living, specifically the Reframing and Mental Rehearsing Tools, I actually like this shot.

her to join, too. "She was very supportive," Sharon recalls. "We both lost the weight and became lifetime members."

Sharon maintained her slimmer status until she had children; afterward, she was left with a legacy of pregnancy weight. Then came another moment of truth: "I saw a picture of myself holding one of my daughters and I was horrified at how heavy I was," she remembers. "I think most of us think of ourselves as being at the last weight we could tolerate, so that's what we see when we look in the mirror. But we could be a lot heavier." Because her stepdaughter had lost 30 pounds through Weight Watchers at the age of 11, and kept the weight off throughout her teen years and later joined the track team, Sharon was convinced that this was a plan that could truly help people such as herself make better choices. Once again, Sharon joined and lost 50 pounds from her 5-foot 4½-inch frame in 1981. "Before that, I didn't really believe I could do it," confesses Sharon, who has four kids in her blended family (her husband was married once before). "I used to say, 'It's too hard.' This time, I decided to pretend this was a pregnancy: I would give myself nine months. And there were times when I'd wonder, 'Why is it taking so long?' or 'This should be over already.' But I stuck with it and it took 10 months."

One of the keys to her success was giving her environment a makeover. It helped that there were three generations of women supporting each other in the weight-loss process, but Sharon also made some changes around the house. "I decided not to have stuff that got me into trouble—ice cream or big bags of chips," she explains. "I got rid of my scale. I threw it out because I was playing games. If I stepped on it and saw it was down two pounds before the end of the week, I'd celebrate and eat. Or, if I went to a wedding and I was good but gained a couple of pounds, I'd eat. The scale wasn't helping me; it was hindering me." (Even now, she weighs herself just once a month. "I can tell how I'm doing by how my clothes fit," she says.)

Sharon also began tinkering with the content of family meals. Rather than having vegetables only as a side dish, the family began eating more vegetables. "We eat huge salads every single night," she explains. "And we have a garden in our yard, where we grow eggplant, zucchini, tomatoes, string beans, cucumbers and herbs." Sharon also began drinking lots of water throughout the day. When making food choices, she'd consider: What can I eat today that's going to make this body look good or keep this body looking the way I want it to look?

Even though she lost weight without exercising, she knew that exercise would have to become part of the maintenance equation at some point. The trouble was, she'd always hated exercise. "About four or five years ago, I realized I needed to exercise to be healthier," she recalls. She and her assistant had a morning ritual of meeting for coffee before work. Sharon suggested an alternative idea: getting together an hour before work for a brisk walk at the mall. "This way we get to catch up with each other and we get our exercise in," says Sharon, who continues to do this four times a week.

To keep herself motivated to eat healthfully while shedding pounds, Sharon relied on mental exercises: "I had a rule: if I wanted to eat something that wasn't on the plan or that wouldn't fit into the program for the day, I would close my eyes and picture what I'd want to look like," she explains. "Then I'd open my eyes and decide if this food would help me get there. Or I'd consider if I could have it and avoid the snowball effect, where I'd keep eating and eating." She also gave herself pep talks to keep herself going: "I tried to say at the end of the day, 'Today was good; tomorrow will be even better,'" Sharon recalls. "The more I'd say it, the more I'd start to believe it." And when the naysayer within would speak up and say something like "Why did you eat that?" Sharon would try to silence her inner critic. "When I did that, I'd try to have an alarm go off in my head and make myself stop," she says. "I'd tell myself to treat myself as nicely as I would a friend or stranger. I'd say, 'Just pick yourself up now.'"

It's sound advice—and it's paid off handsomely for Sharon. "My self-confidence level after losing the weight is so much greater," she says. "I wouldn't do as many things—such as standing in front of a hundred people and talking—as I do now. I certainly like what I see in the mirror better. I like my body better but I also realize the body is just a body. What's inside I feel so much better about. I feel proud of the fact that it's been more than 18 years that I've had the weight off. It makes me feel empowered. Now I try to apply what I've learned to other areas. I'm clearer about what I want and why I want it. It has so much to do with doing things for yourself and getting over your fears. When you try to get past them, sometimes it works and sometimes it doesn't. But it's always a learning process."

Change doesn't happen in a vacuum. It happens in the context of your life, in the circumstances of your world. You can have the best intentions, the highest motivation, and the most effective goal-setting techniques on the planet, but if your environment doesn't support the changes you're trying to make, the self-improvement process will be much harder than it has to be. Just as it can seem nearly impossible to stay healthy when half of your office has a nasty stomach bug, it can be extremely difficult to stick with changes you're making when your environment seems determined to thwart your goals. Yet most people don't even consider the role their environment plays as they pursue their missions. They simply forge ahead, oblivious to the power that physical surroundings can exert on their behavior.

And that's a mistake that can come back to haunt you. Take an unvarnished look at your surroundings and assess what isn't working or what may be hindering your efforts to reach your goals. Do forces that undermine your ambitions lurk around every corner? Is your home set up in such a way that it's difficult for you to locate the tools you need when you need them? To a certain extent you can take steps to modify your surroundings. In fact, research has found that people can alter or restructure their environment in such a way that it will help control their behavior. In a study of pregnant women who were trying to quit smoking, for example, researchers from the University of Texas in Houston looked at what distinguished who was successful from who wasn't. Among the contributing factors: The quitters altered their environment so that it would help them *not* smoke—by throwing away the pack of cigarettes in their purse or by giving themselves a substitute activity when they felt the urge to smoke, for instance.

There's no denying that allowing your environment to support your goals is incredibly helpful when it comes to changing bad habits. But this effect doesn't just apply to your home environment, although that is a large part of it. It also involves your social world, your workplace, and your lifestyle.

In a nutshell, what you want to do is modify *all* of these environments so that it promotes your ability to attain your goals, instead of working against you or presenting additional, unnecessary obstacles. For example, if having a drink causes you to snack or smoke (and you're trying to kick this habit), you could structure your schedule so that going to happy hour after work becomes impossible.

If you're trying to muster every ounce of energy and enthusiasm you can for an upcoming challenge, you could choose to temporarily limit your contact with family members who are energy vampires. You can also set up your environment so that it *promotes* a behavior you're trying to cultivate, by making a date to meet friends at the gym after work if you're trying to become an exercise devotee, for instance. And finally, you can arrange your environment so that it continuously reminds you of your goals without nagging you. You could keep your gym bag by the front door. You could post affirmations above your desk at work or you could place a stop sign or a photo of your once-slim self in a bikini on the door to the refrigerator.

In short, you want to learn to control your environment so that it no longer controls you. This is yet another example of a proactive approach to the self-improvement process—and it's a powerful one. Environmental control can help you remove things from your home or office that promote the behavior you're trying to kick, and it can give you the power to stay away from places or people that encourage exactly what you don't want to do. It also lets you place positive reminders throughout your surroundings that will inspire you to keep embracing the changes you're making. It's making your world work with you instead of against you, which will make striving for your goals that much easier and less frustrating. This, in turn, will improve the odds that you'll stick with the process.

Places of Influence

Most of us spend the majority of our time either at home or at work. And while your home may be your haven, that doesn't mean it is set up to help you achieve your personal goals. The same could be said for the workplace:

Giving Your Surroundings
a Weight-Related Makeover

This may be the perfect time to redecorate your home. Not literally. But you can revamp your surroundings so that they promote more of the behavior that you're trying to cultivate and discourage the habits and patterns you're trying to bid farewell to. How? By making a list of environmental qualities that would further your goals and then taking inventory of your home, room by room.

In the kitchen, consider:

Stocking your pantry and fridge with healthy foods. You can't change your eating habits unless you change the food you have around, so out with the junk food and in with the healthy stuff. Fill your fridge with fresh fruits, vegetables, skim milk, low-fat mayonnaise and salad dressings, low-fat cheeses and yogurt, fresh fish and other wholesome fare. Load up your pantry with low-fat whole-grain crackers, pasta, brown rice, canned beans and vegetables, whole-grain cereals, dried fruits (raisins, cranberries, cherries), low-fat soups, flavored vinegars (to use instead of oils), water-packed tuna and reduced-fat microwave popcorn (for snacks). Your body will thank you.

Making the good stuff accessible. Keep a bowl of fresh fruit on the counter, and if your schedule is hectic, consider keeping prewashed, precut vegetables in the fridge.

Keeping your measuring cups and spoons in plain view. Do the same with a food scale, if you use one. By moving these items out from the shadows of the cabinet, you'll be more likely to put them to use when measuring your portions.

Placing a mirror on the wall. A recent study from Iowa State Uni-

continued on next page

versity in Ames found that people who ate in a room with a mirror ate considerably less regular cream cheese or margarine on their bagels. The theory is that when people focus attention on themselves, they become aware of any discrepancies between their actual behavior and their goals.

In the bedroom, consider:

Hanging a full-length mirror. Instead of having to guess what you look like, you'll be able see a realistic reflection. And you'll be able to see progress in how your clothes fit. After embarking on a weight-loss plan, it takes about six weeks for clothes to start fitting differently. Once that begins to happen, you'll probably experience a renewed sense of motivation to continue.

Placing your exercise gear and shoes in plain view. This will serve as a gentle reminder to get moving on a regular basis.

In the bathroom, consider:

Getting rid of the scale. It doesn't always tell the truth about what's going on in your body. If you step on the scale a few days before your period arrives, you might think you've gained weight when it's really just temporary water retention. Or, if you begin exercising more, particularly if you add strength training on a regular basis, you might wind up losing body fat (which takes up more space but weighs less) and gaining muscle mass (which takes up less space but weighs more). Instead, consider keeping a tape measure handy so that you can measure how many inches you've lost.

It's the setting where you're supposed to be productive and efficient, but that doesn't necessarily mean that you are. The truth is, all kinds of subtle traps exist in both settings, potholes that can trip you up as you pursue your goals. Some of them may be plainly visible, others are less obvious.

As you examine your surroundings, ask yourself the following questions: What, if anything, in this environment could impede my progress toward my goals? What forces could be at work here that could undermine my resolve when it's shaky? What could I bring to this environment that would serve as positive reinforcement as I pursue my goals?

Let's say you're trying to lose weight: If your pantry is filled with chips, cookies and other high-fat, high-sugar snack foods, that's a blatant example of how your environment—in this case, the temptations it contains—could hinder your efforts. If your fridge is fully stocked, except for break-fast foods, that's a subtler snare, because eating a healthy breakfast can help you stick with healthy eating habits all day long. And, finally, if fresh pro-duce is conspicuously absent from your kitchen, that's another way in which your environment isn't serving your best interests. The same is true if you put yourself in the position of having to turn to a vending machine if you get hungry at work; that's why it's smart to keep a few healthy snacks—single servings of pretzels, individual boxes of dry cereal or raisins, cups of soup and the like—stashed in a desk drawer.

By the same token, if you're launching a search from home for a more gratifying job, your environment can help you, if a game plan is in plain view on your home-office desk. Or it could hinder you, if your desk is such a mess that you can't find anything when you need it.

Letting your environment support your goals can have a softer touch, too. You probably realize that placing feel-good objects—whether it's a fa-vorite art piece, a family photograph, or some other kind of trinket—on display in your home can positively influence your state of mind. But this psychological boost can indirectly support your goals, too, especially if it serves as a reminder of your essential values.

Similarly, if you have a highly stressful job, placing photographs of scenes of nature or even potted plants in your office could ease the strain. Research has found that nature can relieve what psychologists call "mental fatigue," an inner weariness and an inability to concentrate that can set in after an intense period of hard work that consumes lots of focused atten-tion. But the big surprise is that you don't have to go into the wild to reap these benefits. Studies have found that people whose offices have views of trees and flowers typically feel less pressured and more satisfied with their jobs. What's more, a study in a suburban Pennsylvania hospital found that patients whose rooms looked out on a natural setting had shorter postoperative stays, earned fewer negative comments in nurses' notes, and took less pain medication than patients whose windows faced a brick wall. If you don't have a room with a view at work, don't worry: Simply give yourself a natural scene to look at by hanging posters or pictures near your desk.

Of course, it also helps to place positive reminders of your goals around your environment—by putting your jogging clothes and shoes at your bedside if you're trying to exercise each morning, or posting a "Do It Now!" sign above your desk if you want to stop procrastinating or a sign that says "Work Smarter" if you want to improve your efficiency at the office. What's important is that you choose a reminder that resonates for you. Basically, positive reminders serve two purposes: One, they act almost like a "pause" button in the midst of a busy day; they force you to stop and consider what's in your best interest to do. And, second, they function almost like visual pep talks that are designed to spur you into action. Either way, they can help you stay on the right track to your goals.

The Social Arena

Be forewarned: Some people in your life may not be happy with your efforts to improve yourself or your quality of life. Like it or not, we all have a "Board of Advisers," a group of people who, often tacitly, influence our values and goals. We may not have chosen them but there they are. These people, your family and friends, often preserve the status quo, encouraging us to stay within our comfort zones.

If your goals go against the grain of their values and perspectives, people around you might find your effort to change threatening because it disrupts their comfort zone, because they're afraid you might outgrow them, or because it calls their own values into question. As a result, they may, consciously or not, attempt to sabotage your efforts to change by saying things like "Just this once . . ." or "It's too hard to change . . ." Others may simply encourage the behavior you're trying to kick by planning or organizing activities that promote it.

As a starting point, you can try to reason with these people or try to reassure them that your efforts to change won't affect your relationship—and that may make a difference. It also may help to try to incorporate them into your plans, by inviting a friend you used to meet for lunch to come work out with you at the gym (if you're trying to slim down), or by inviting a colleague who has become a close friend to attend a networking seminar with you (if you're trying to land a new job).

But if their sabotaging ways get out of hand, there may come a time when you could face an unpleasant choice—between them and your own growth and well-being. If you're really committed to attaining your goals, spending time with people who don't support your efforts may not be as appealing as it once was. So if you generally eat or drink too much when you go out with your college buddies and you're trying to lose weight or lead a healthier life, you might decide to stop hanging out with them for a while. Similarly, if you often take a midafternoon break to go out for coffee and cookies with colleagues, you might prefer to take a brisk walk with an exercise buddy instead.

And if you're trying to cultivate a more upbeat, proactive approach toward life in general, you may not want to spend time with someone who continually drags down your mood or disparages your efforts to change. After all, there are people who fuel your energy with their upbeat attitudes and loving, appreciative spirits—and people who can make it fizzle with their constant complaining and negativity. When you look at it this way, whom would you prefer to be around?

Ideally, you'll want to find allies who can support the changes you're trying to make, and you might be surprised when you discover them in the most unlikely places. Sometimes the friends and family members you expect to be the most supportive of your quest for self-improvement let you down. But often other people on whom you don't usually rely, will come through for you and boost your efforts in the most helpful ways. To find these people, sometimes all it takes is to go public with your goals by telling friends, family members, colleagues and neighbors what you're trying to achieve. Think of yourself as a magnet, trying to draw positive people toward you who can buoy your resolve, share the secrets behind their skills and success, and challenge you to become the best you that you

The Importance of Social Support

Changing your life is hard, but it becomes even harder if you take the solo route. Gathering support from family, friends and colleagues, on the other hand, can really boost your odds of succeeding.

For example, in a study of participants enrolled in a low-calorie diet and behavior modification program at a Rhode Island hospital, those who were able to maintain their weight loss two years later credited a maintenance support group, among other factors, as helping them. Researchers at Stanford University discovered that social support—especially from family and friends—was a strong predictor of adherence to an exercise program for 269 women and men.

Why is support so vital? It's partly because we're social creatures. We like being with other people, as well as earning their encouragement, praise and recognition when we succeed. The people you turn to for support can also help remind you of what's worked for you in the past and what hasn't—and how to keep things in perspective when your willpower crumbles. Checking in with others regularly can help you stay on the right track. Here's how to make the most of your own support group.

Find the system that works for you. Not every system works for everybody, so it's important to work out an arrangement that makes sense for you. If you can't see yourself speaking up in a group, don't join one. Consider working with a personal coach or a buddy instead.

Be direct about your needs and goals. Be specific about how you'd like others to support you; don't expect them to read your mind. Tell members of your support network what they can say or do that will be most helpful to you. Rather than ask someone

continued on next page

to monitor your behavior, which could make you feel like rebelling, it's more helpful to have someone to talk to when you're suffering motivational crises or someone who can give you perspective or advice about your behavior when you're struggling.

Fess up about what's really going on. Honesty really is the best policy when it comes to your habits. Otherwise, you'll be giving your support system a skewed or partial picture of the obstacles you're facing, in which case they won't really know how to help you.

Make your arrangement official. If you decide to work with a buddy, formalize how often you'll check in with each other and when, and think of contingency plans. These days, most people have such jam-packed schedules that unless you make an appointment to talk, it may not happen. If your buddy is not available, it can turn into an excuse for falling away from the plan. In those instances, you need to have a backup activity in mind or someone else you can turn to in a pinch.

Show appreciation to those who've helped you. And try to reciprocate in some way. Not only does giving back feel good, but acknowledging, thanking and rewarding people for the support you've come to rely on is the best way of ensuring that it continues.

can be. Once you have this inner circle of trusted allies—your new, personally appointed Board of Advisers—don't be afraid to turn to them when you need their help or support.

Identifying Your Danger Zones

It doesn't matter how much willpower or determination you have: Everybody is vulnerable to lapses in certain situations despite his or her good intentions. But what triggers that crisis of control for one person may be quite different from what does it for someone else. That's why it's important to zero in on *your* danger zones. Look around you and ask yourself: In what settings am I most likely to engage in the behavior I'm trying to kick? Are there people in my life who have contributed to the continuation of this unwanted behavior, whether it's overeating or being passive at work, and, if so, who are they?

The idea isn't to find a way to cast blame; that's a waste of time and energy. What you want to do instead is to pinpoint the times and places when it will be especially difficult for you to act in accordance with your goals. Once you know where trouble lies for you, it's smart to do whatever you can—within reason—to help yourself avoid or minimize your contact with the circumstances, geographical places and people in your life that encourage you to stay within the comfort zone of old, unwanted behavior, at least until you've established new, improved habits. In the meantime, it's better to set yourself up for success by replacing the downward push of negative influences with the upward pull of supportive ones.

But there will come a point when it's not possible for you to avoid things that trigger a form of behavior that you're trying to put in the past. And when the trigger is right in front of you, you'll have to find a way to deal with it effectively so that you can triumph over temptation or avoid lapsing into a less desirable form of behavior. Remember: *While you may not be able to change a particular situation, you can control your response to it.*

One way to do this is to desensitize yourself mentally and emotionally to the trigger factor by confronting it in your imagination ahead of time. Visualize yourself meeting the challenge head-on and coming up with an effective response. If you're trying to lose weight and you know you'll be going to an extended family get-together that will be chock-full of food pushers, it may help to imagine yourself firmly saying, "No, thank you," again and again ahead of time. This way, you won't hesitate when you're actually in that situation. Similarly, if you're trying to cultivate a more composed attitude at work and you'll be going on a company retreat with your tense, demanding boss, practice deep-breathing exercises while you imagine him spouting off; when the time comes, you'll have a greater chance of keeping your cool.

Time Management 101

Let's dispel this notion from the very beginning: There is no such thing as "free time" and there never will be. Large chunks of unused time don't magically appear out of nowhere—and no one will hand you extra hours in any given day or week. Time is a precious commodity, and many of us perpetually feel as though we don't have enough time to do everything we have to do, as though we don't have a moment to spare. This means that if you want to find the time it takes to engage effectively in the planning and activities that are involved in pursuing your goals, you're going to have to *make* the time. And that means you're going to have to carve it out of what is probably already a busy life. It *is* possible to do this.

After all, how you choose to spend your time is ultimately up to you. And if you're going to revamp your life, you may need to restructure how you use your time. But first, you'll need to get an accurate assessment of where your time actually goes. The best way to do that is to act like a lawyer and account for every minute of your time. Keep a time log for two or three days and track how you spend every five-minute block. Then tally up the minutes and divide what consumes your time and attention into the following categories: sleeping, eating, actually working (as opposed to simply being at work), socializing with friends or colleagues, spending time with your spouse or family, leisure activity (reading, hobbies), taking care of personal business (your home, errands, laundry), watching television, taking care of yourself (relaxing, grooming, exercising), community work, religious or spiritual activity, and time that's unaccounted for. You may be surprised at where you're actually spending your time.

After you've completed this reality check, reassess how you'd like to be spending your time. Maybe you'll discover that you have an hour a day that's unaccounted for and you might decide that you'd like to harness this time and spend it by taking a class, spending more quality time with your spouse or engaging in a spiritual pursuit. Maybe you'll realize that you're spending more time than you'd like to eating or watching TV and you could spend this time taking better care of your health and well-being. The idea is to manage your time so that it accurately reflects your new priorities and allows you to pursue your goals rather than letting your time manage you.

The key is to be willing to set personal priorities, establish limits with other people, say no to requests or invitations that are a drain on your time and energy, and delegate tasks that aren't essential for you to do. If you're not clear about what your priorities are in your job, you should sit down with your supervisor and discuss this. You can do the same thing on the home front: Discuss with your spouse and other family members what activities they perceive to be the most important. You might discover that they'd rather eat frozen dinners a couple of nights each week and have more quality time with you. Or someone else in the family might volunteer to help you with the laundry or another chore to give you more leisure time at home.

Once you're clear about your priorities, you'll need to get into the habit of scheduling your time the way you want to. The best way to do this is to keep a calendar or a day planner and to devote the bulk of your time to the activities, duties and interests that you've designated as the most important in your life. Ideally, you should make a list of the tasks you want to accomplish every day and mark these A, B or C, depending on their relative importance, so that you are absolutely certain about what it is you should be doing with your time. Start with the A list, then proceed to the B, and so on. If you perform specific activities every day, such as exercising, try to do them at the same time each day to take the guesswork out of having to find a time slot.

But remember: Everything usually takes slightly longer than you think it will. So build in a grace period, add a little maneuvering room to your schedule to prevent yourself from becoming overscheduled and perpetually crunched for time. If you think you can complete a report in three days of work, give yourself four, to be on the safe side. If you think you can review a friend's creative plan by Wednesday, promise that you'll get back to her by the end of the week, just in case something unexpected comes up. In fact, time-management experts often recommend keeping at least a 60-minute window open each day to deal with unexpected events or crises. By building a little breathing room into your schedule, you'll be allowing yourself to proceed with the expected stuff at a sane pace, which can add to the enjoyment of what you're doing, and you'll be boosting your odds of meeting deadlines, which will enhance your reputation for reliability.

Taking the time to plan out your daily activities in advance may seem counterproductive in terms of time management, since it eats up time. But the minutes you invest in performing this task up front—it shouldn't take more than 10 to 15 minutes—will bring a larger return later in the day. It will actually make more time available throughout the day because it will spell out exactly what needs to get done and make your use of time more efficient. As a result, it will eliminate all that wasted time you normally spend thinking about what you should be doing next.

Get Organized

It's not just a matter of making your environment look tidier and less cluttered. Arranging things in an orderly manner can actually improve your efficiency. It helps you avoid having to spend time needlessly looking for the items you require to function. And this, in turn, can make you feel less stressed and less harried. Getting organized is really about identifying what matters to you and making sure that it's accessible. Although the challenge is to find a system that works for you, there are certain organizing principles that seem to work for most people. Here are four that have wide applications throughout your life:

Set up workable systems.

Rule number one is to make sure that everything has its own designated place. At home, that means keeping your checkbook and bank statements in one spot, perhaps in a drawer in a desk or secretary. Place keys on a rack in the kitchen, in a hallway, or by the door. Put your purse in the same place—on a hook in the coat closet or on a counter in the kitchen for example—when you're not using it. By taking these steps, you'll save yourself the time and aggravation of having to comb your home looking for these items when you need them. You can use the same technique to or-

Improving Your Odds by Design

Wouldn't it be great if you could change your life just by re-arranging your furniture? Well, it's not quite that easy, but it's close, at least according to the ancient Chinese art of placement and design known as *feng shui* (pronounced *fung schway*). The basic principle is to manipulate your physical surroundings in order to nudge your destiny in a favorable direction. The idea is that correct placement of furniture, mirrors, plants and colors, as well as proper use of your living space, can improve the flow of *chi* (or vital energy) throughout your home, putting you in a more harmonious position with nature and the universe.

Does this sound like magic? It's actually more like a cross between art and science, philosophy and superstition. But properly used, feng shui is believed to have a positive influence on your attitude, your personal energy, even on the most intimate details of your private and professional life. Perhaps that's why the discipline is gaining popularity in the United States. Fortunately, many of feng shui's principles can easily be put into practice in your home. What follows are five ways to improve energy circulation and hence the flow of good luck throughout your home.

Use all the burners on your stove regularly, instead of relying on just one or two. The theory is that this can enhance your family's income potential by allowing heat and energy to pass continuously through each of these openings. Also, make sure the stove is always kept clean to ensure the family's good health (the buildup of grease can supposedly create problems because it's an example of neglecting proper hygiene).

Reposition your bed so that you can see the doorway. Being startled by a visitor can supposedly disrupt your *chi*. If the room doesn't

continued on next page

allow this, placing a mirror on the wall so that it reflects the doorway will also do the trick.

Choose soft, pastel-colored towels for your bathroom to promote good health and cash flow. Green is a restful color that is believed to aid digestion, whereas blue, which is associated with bodies of water, will supposedly discourage plumbing problems and encourage financial prosperity.

Place a plant or a bouquet of red flowers in the marriage area of a room—which happens to be in the far right corner from the door—to keep your marriage flourishing. Plants symbolize growth, freshness and tranquility; red is considered an auspicious color.

Keep hallways unobstructed so that energy and opportunities can flow freely into each room. The same goes for doorways. By keeping these spaces open, the theory is that you won't constrict your potential for personal growth.

ganize your use of time at home: Designate Saturday morning as grocery-shopping time; Monday night might be your chosen time for paying bills. Being consistent in your organizational habits can help you use time more efficiently.

Arrange your environment sensibly.

At work, organize your desk so that the items you use every day are within arm's reach. Those that are needed less frequently—say, once a month—should be placed in a file cabinet or in storage. Use folders to organize To Do items (lists of reminders, letters to be answered, and so on) as well as To Be Filed items (things you want to hold on to but won't need for a while or things you haven't decided what to do with).

You can employ similar strategies at home. In your kitchen, you might keep the seasonings you use regularly within reach of the stove on a spice rack and those you use less often in a cabinet. You can also create a filing system for household business—a To Do folder with bills to pay and a To Be Filed folder for family medical records, insurance claims, auto and home insurance statements and so on.

Become an expert at multitasking.

Basically, this means try to do more than one thing at a time whenever possible. Fold the laundry while you're catching up on phone calls to friends and relatives. Use your commute time (if you're not driving, that is) to read the paper or to pen your daily To Do list. Prepare dinner while you supervise your kids doing their homework. Once again, this adds up to efficient use of your time.

Schedule time on a regular basis for reorganizing.

Give yourself an hour or two once a week to go through your To Do and To Be Filed folders and either trash what's no longer needed or deal with what you've fallen behind on. Retrieve any stray items that aren't where they belong and put them in their place.

Taking these steps to organize your life may seem incredibly mundane when you can be thinking about improving your life on a much higher level. But they're necessary. For one thing, creating order in your day-to-day existence frees up your mind and your energy for more important pursuits. It also allows you to use your time more efficiently in general, and it might even make more time available for your goal-related activities by sparing you from the hassle of having to locate the things you need in a chaotic environment. As the eighteenth-century Irish statesman Edmund Burke once noted, "Good order is the foundation of all good things." With a solid foundation supporting you, you'll be able to build a sturdier house of dreams.

ASSIGNMENT Map out a support network like a family tree. Start with those who are closest to home (i.e., your immediate family), then branch out to those who belong to your extended family, your circle of friends, your neighbors, your colleagues from work and so on. Once you've got a detailed picture of who belongs to your support network, use different colors of pen to highlight which people you would turn to for advice on how to pursue your goals, whom you would turn to for moral support, who would be especially helpful if you were to suffer a crisis of confidence and so on. By creating an illustration of this network, you'll probably come to realize that you have a treasure trove of support right at your disposal whenever you need it.

CHAPTER SEVEN

Becoming a Friend to Yourself

*I*magine having a lovely room in your home that goes unused because it's meant only for special guests. You invite a friend over and suddenly there you are fluffing the pillows, arranging flowers, lighting candles and laying out your best tea. You want to make your friend feel welcome and special and of course all these little preparations will do just that.

Do you think others should fuss over you? More important, would you fuss for yourself? If little acts of kindness are the basis of good friendships, then it stands to reason that we need to honor ourselves with supportive words and gestures. Many of us don't do unto ourselves as we do to others, and I can tell you it's a mistake. I would have been a lot of happier if I had. We need to start doing it because, let's face it, who else will do it for us? As my grandma used to tell me, "Give a smile and receive a smile." Take compliments, for example. Much of my life I've deflected compliments as if accepting one would be immodest or egotistical. I learned at such an early age not to be selfish because Dads told me not to be that way. Selfish is to talk about myself and to have any consideration for myself. So I grew up thinking I was selfish and gradually became my own harshest judge. Now I am beginning to learn that I might do things that are okay, that I might be a nice person, and I am starting to get much better at accepting praise, but I have a way to go.

Lucy Lonning, the Weight Watchers leader featured in this chapter, reminds me of the parlor that's only good enough for guests. Lucy told me about how she felt ridiculed and humiliated as a child because she was overweight. She said she compensated for the hurt by being a perfectionist and by going overboard to win people's approval. Lucy recalls baking birthday cakes for everyone in high school, hoping it would make her more likable. Her low self-esteem only perpetuated the pattern of excessive giving right into adulthood, though, and when she felt overwhelmed, Lucy would eat to procrastinate, regardless of the consequences.

Weight Watchers was like a fresh start for Lucy because it gave her a game plan that allowed her to call the shots. She quickly learned to visualize her goal of wearing smaller clothes and at one point even hung a beautiful new skirt outside her closet for inspiration. The discipline that came with establishing new eating habits also helped Lucy live in the present. As the pounds came off, Lucy had a more positive outlook on life, and this extended to how she thought about herself. She finally set limits with other people at work, in relationships and with her family, too. To this day Lucy makes maintaining the precious friendship she found within a high priority.

Many of us needlessly cling to painful memories in ways that make the hurt keep on hurting us. A friend at Weight Watchers once gave me a powerful analogy that put this into perspective. "You can't drive a car with your eyes fixed on the rearview mirror," she said. Although my friend truly believed in what she said and I must agree with her to a great extent, I might add that even today, at the ripe young age of 41, there are still days when I look back with deep regret at some of my past behavior and actions. I think I always will. It's just me and I'm just human. And the lesson I've learned here is that I can embrace that part of me as well.

Profile: **LUCY LONNING**
Becoming a Friend to Myself

Lucy Lonning went on her first diet in seventh grade, back when unkind classmates called her Moose. In the years that followed, she tried just about every fad diet known to man- and womankind. First, there were the Stillman, the Atkins, and the Scarsdale diets, the U.S. Ski Team diet, and even the cab-

bage soup diet; then she joined several weight-loss programs. Her mother was also overweight, so often the two would diet together. When Lucy was in high school, her mother began going to Weight Watchers and Lucy asked to go with her; her mother said no, largely because she didn't want her daughter to know what she weighed. So Lucy was left to her own weight-loss devices, and no matter what she tried, she couldn't seem to lose weight permanently.

"Over the years, I've been up and down 55 pounds, with my highest weight in college," recalls Lucy, now 45, a Weight Watchers leader in Connecticut. (At one point, she was wearing size 38 men's jeans. "I pretended I was buying them for my brother," she quips.) "I was always an emotional eater and a procrastination eater. I always have so much to do—a list 10 yards long—that it's overwhelming. So I would eat to procrastinate, to put off getting started, and it could go on all day. I'd eat anything, but especially carbohydrates."

Lucy didn't quite realize the toll this habit was taking on her 5-foot 10-inch figure until the summer of 1988. That's when she took three trips and managed to gain weight on each one. "When I saw a picture of myself on one of those trips, I decided to lose weight," she says. "I wasn't comfortable meeting new people. I was worried that they wouldn't like me because I wasn't attractive."

Because she had a friend who was a lifetime member of Weight Watchers, she decided to join. "Once I got started, it seemed so possible to me," she says. "I wanted to fit into smaller sizes so I took a beautiful Evan Picone wool skirt and hung it up against the closet for inspiration. I never put it away. I wanted to wear that by the end of the winter." Keeping this goal constantly in her sights encouraged Lucy to revamp some of her habits. "Because I live alone, I used to have vegetables in the house only when company came, but I realized that I like vegetables," she notes. "And I became addicted to the energy I got from eating healthfully. I didn't consciously say, 'I have to eat better for me.' But within a couple of weeks, I started feeling different. I had more energy; it was easier to get out of bed; I didn't get tired as easily during the day; I could stay up and be clear-minded into the evening."

To this day, though, Lucy doesn't deprive herself of what she really wants. If she craves chocolate (she's a self-described chocoholic) or tacos from a fast-food joint, she simply finds a way to fit these indulgences into her overall plan. Another big change: becoming an exercise devotee. "I used to exercise in spurts," Lucy confesses. "Now I walk every day for about half an hour. And I really do feel weird when I don't get it in. I don't have as much energy when I don't get a walk."

Though she hasn't completely kicked the procrastination-eating habit, Lucy has found ways to minimize the damage. "When I notice I'm doing it, I don't allow myself to eat until I've gotten one of the projects done or I set up times when I'm allowed to eat," she explains. Likewise, when her emotional keel tilts off balance, she has learned to find other ways to handle her feelings—by knitting ("which is repetitive and soothing"), playing with her two English setters or gardening.

After Lucy lost 32 pounds and reached her goal in 1989, she became a full-time Weight Watchers leader and now runs 13 meetings a week. She also lost a lot of emotional distress by learning to treat herself more kindly. "When I lost all the weight, I went to a workshop about discovering yourself and learning from the past. I've eased up on my expectations of myself and I've learned how to forgive myself. I was definitely a black-and-white-person: If I was off (in my diet) in the morning, I was off for the whole day. It was always perfectionist thinking. It makes your life so much easier when you realize you don't have to be 100 percent all the time; when you realize the house looks good enough, that it doesn't have to be perfect.

"Once you can learn to say 'Oh, well' or 'I'm only human' and let it go, it's a real relief," she says. "I learned to do this when I realized I lost my weight without being perfect. One slip isn't going to get in your way when it comes to losing weight; the one thing you say to your boss isn't going to get you fired; or the bad thing you say to a family member isn't going to mean the end of the relationship. If you can't go back and change it, it's important to move on. All days are good days; some days are just better than others. I think we all have cycles; some are more up than others. But even in the down cycles, you have to look around and see the good stuff. It's there—you just have to focus on what you do have."

In the process of shedding pounds and unrealistic expectations, Lucy adopted a more philosophical attitude toward life. That shift encouraged her to be less critical of herself and to treat herself as if she were her own good friend. And this, in turn, has increased her willingness to make her own well-being a top priority and to set limits with other people—at work, in relationships and with her family. "Losing weight freed me up to be who I was all the time," she says. "I used to hide behind the weight. I always knew I was smart and funny but I didn't have the self-confidence to *get involved with other people or in different activities. Now I can go to parties or I can talk to people in stores because I think of myself as a normal person.*

"For me, the biggest change was letting go of the fantasy that someday this knight in shining armor would come along and take care of me," she adds. "I realized I didn't need or want that. So I bought a house for myself instead of waiting for a husband to come along. I feel good enough about me to take chances and do things I want to do. I'm not waiting for things to happen."

OUR INNER THOUGHTS can be our best friends or our worst enemies. Think about all the times you've given yourself a pep talk and then felt much more confident and competent. Or how focusing on all the things that could go right—rather than wrong—when a job change helped you take smart chances that paid off. Now consider the times you've sabotaged your own emotional well-being in subtle ways. Maybe a little voice inside your head told you that you were fat before you went to a pool party. Or maybe you sent yourself on a first-class guilt trip when you went away for a romantic weekend with your spouse and left the kids at Grandma's house.

Many of us hold ourselves to impossible standards, judging ourselves much more harshly than we would a friend. Not only is this counterproductive but it becomes a habit that can take a toll on your self-esteem and can even lead to depression or anxiety. On the other hand, if you make a conscious effort to start treating yourself with the tenderness, care and consideration that you would your dearest friends, you can bolster your self-esteem and your emotional well-being. And this, in turn, can help you achieve your goals. If this positive style doesn't come naturally, you can make the shift by giving your interior world a makeover.

After all, when it comes to making meaningful changes or striving to improve your life, attitude is nearly everything. This orientation of the mind is the filter through which every event and encounter in your life passes. Without your ability to experience and process the world around you, the world would not exist for you. You see the world through your own eyes, and you interpret it and give it meaning with your perceptions. In other words, your observations, thoughts and beliefs create your reality. And it's your thoughts and attitudes that drive your intentions and goals, which, in turn, direct your behavior. So if you want to alter your behavior or improve your performance, it makes sense to start at the beginning of the chain reaction—by changing your mind-set. After all, how you act in life is often a reflection of your inner thoughts and beliefs. It really is the thoughts that count.

Giving Yourself an Attitude Check

While you're immersed in the process of change or the pursuit of new goals, you may begin to recognize certain patterns to the messages that float through your mind. These patterns stem from your basic attitudes and beliefs, which are deeply rooted and have a profound influence on nearly every aspect of your life.

To a large extent, your attitudes and beliefs about a given situation or event will determine how you experience it. If you're like most people, you basically trust your beliefs to be true, so you aren't likely to challenge them; you probably just accept them at face value and act accordingly. Yet your perceptions and interpretations, which basically combine to create your beliefs, can be skewed versions of what's really going on. If you need evidence of this, just consider how different various people's versions of the same event can be when they describe it. Each person perceives reality in a slightly different way based on her attitudes and beliefs—and none is necessarily completely accurate.

There's a problem, however, if your beliefs are based on erroneous assumptions or negative attitudes, because then they can hold you back from accomplishing your goals. So if you're vying for a promotion at work or striving to lose weight or competing in an athletic event, and you're carrying around a grab bag of beliefs that tell you that you won't be able to do it, you're pretty much destined to fail before you even start.

That's why it's important to identify the self-limiting beliefs that could be restraining you, and challenge and correct them. Self-limiting beliefs can be as varied as the people they belong to, but certain themes generally crop up again and again. Take a look at the following list and see if any of these sound familiar to you:

Common Self-Limiting Beliefs

- I need to feel well loved and secure in my relationships in order to love myself.
- Other people are better than I am at most things in life.
- If I don't live up to other people's expectations, they won't like me.
- I shouldn't make mistakes; I should be perfect.
- People wouldn't like me if they knew the real me.
- I've gotten where I am mostly on luck, not skill.
- I don't deserve to be happy.
- Life is supposed to be fair.
- I am a victim of circumstances that are beyond my control.
- Taking time for myself is selfish.
- I'm too young to rise up the company ladder.
- I'm too old to try a new sport or learn a new skill.
- I don't possess what it takes to succeed in today's world.
- My problems are different from other people's.
- Nothing I do is ever quite good enough.

If these don't ring true for you, think of a few self-limiting beliefs that could be squelching your potential and write them down on a piece of paper or in your journal.

The good news is, you can reclaim control over your beliefs, even the self-defeating ones; you can reframe situations or events in a more positive or constructive light. How? By doing a reality check. If you typically tell yourself that your problems are different from everybody else's, you might point out that you can't possibly know this to be true; after all, you don't have access to other people's innermost thoughts, so how could you possibly know how they think and feel about *their* problems? Similarly, if you've been telling yourself that you're too old to try a new sport, ask yourself, Who says? and point out that it's never too late to try anything—until you're dead.

Basically, whenever you hear one of these self-limiting beliefs being voiced in your head, you'll want to stop what you're doing and challenge it by asking yourself: What's at the root of this belief? What proof is there that it's true? How does continuing to buy into this belief affect my life? What might happen if I stopped?

Another way to eliminate self-defeating attitudes is to confront your worst fears directly in your imagination. If you've been operating under the belief that other people won't like you if you don't live up to their expectations, you might ask yourself: What if the people who had such lofty expectations of me did stop liking me? How would I cope with that? You might realize in the course of examining all the possibilities that this would be more of a reflection on them, suggesting that they don't truly value your friendship or even appreciate you for who you are. And if that's the case, you might ask yourself why you would want to be friends with people like that, anyway. In the end, you might just discover that the worst-case scenario isn't so bad, after all.

Not only will performing this exercise help you feel better right away—because it releases you from the tyranny of unrealistic or irrational beliefs—it can also help you cultivate a healthier belief system that will make you emotionally stronger in the future. By modifying your beliefs, you'll be giving your life a new shape because you'll be setting yourself up to react to it differently. If one thing is true in life, it's this: You may not be able to control what happens—or what other people do or say—but you can guide how you interpret and respond to those events. That alone can make an enormous difference.

Making this psychological shift will allow you to drop the heavy baggage you've been toting around all these years; once you're free of the burden of self-defeating attitudes, the world seems more open. More opportunities present themselves; more things seem possible. You'll be working with yourself, instead of against yourself. And people won't seem as superior or intimidating as perhaps they once did. In short, you'll be on your way to leading a happier life.

Don't Get Mad; Get Back on an Even Keel

It's no secret that emotions can create some of the biggest obstacles along the journey to self-improvement. When researchers at the Massachusetts Institute of Technology surveyed people about their tendency to overeat when under stress, for example, they found that anger, exhaustion, depression and boredom were especially powerful triggers among women. Unbridled emotions can also lead people astray from other lifestyle changes and goals (such as career aspirations). Exhaustion, depression and boredom may pose a particular threat to perseverance: Someone who is overwhelmed by these emotions may be tempted simply to quit her plan of action.

Anger, on the other hand, can do even worse damage. In fact, a study from Case Western Reserve University in Cleveland found that bad moods that were accompanied by high arousal—as in the case of anger, not sadness—were linked with an increase in self-defeating behavior such as thoughtless risk-taking. The theory is that anger does this by impairing an individual's ability to regulate or control herself. No wonder it can be such a destructive force in the process of change.

Without a doubt, anger is one of the most complicated emotions—and one of the most difficult for women to deal with. This is largely a result of how we've been brought up. Chances are, as a child, you probably rarely saw your mother or other women in your family lose their temper. You may have been chastised for getting angry yourself. While it's considered socially acceptable for women to feel sad or depressed or even to cry, angry women are often thought of as inappropriate, aggressive or unattractive. They're often labeled as shrews—or worse. As a result, many women never learn to recognize or handle anger effectively, which can lead to self-sabotaging behavior such as overeating.

Studies have found that women's anger tends to stem from three sources, according to the Women's Anger Research Project at the University of Tennessee in Knoxville: a sense of powerlessness at not being able to change a situation or a person; a sense of injustice involving sexism, racism, manipulation or betrayal; and irresponsible behavior among the people a woman depends on, whether they're friends, colleagues or family members.

The problem is, when anger isn't channeled constructively it usually erupts suddenly or is suppressed; either way, it can have a detrimental effect on your health, your relationships and your weight. Not only can anger increase a woman's risk of developing heart disease, hypertension or cancer, as well as suppressing her immune system, it can also lead to depression and a host of physical ailments such as headaches and stomach troubles. Moreover, the relationship between anger and eating is complex: Not knowing how to calm your anger can send you to the fridge or pantry, seeking to numb uncomfortable or frightening feelings. But gaining weight can also fuel a woman's ire, which can, in turn, increase your tendency to eat for emotional reasons. In fact, researchers from the University of Pittsburgh recently found that high anger and hostility levels, as measured on standardized tests, were associated with central obesity (the so-called apple-shaped pattern of weight gain) in healthy postmenopausal women; central obesity is known to be an important risk factor for chronic disease, particularly heart disease.

So what can you do instead of swallowing your anger in the form of food? Try these defusing tactics:

Keep an anger journal

Whenever you feel your temper rising, rate your anger on a 10-point scale; if it's a 4 or higher, describe the situation including images and thoughts that come to mind, how long your anger lasts, and the short- and long-term consequences of your explosive feelings. By doing this, you can begin to see patterns in your responses and behavior. If your anger rates a 3 or lower, try to envision it leaving your body and mind in a puff of smoke. It's just not worth it to sweat the little things.

Practice relaxing under pressure.

When you have some free time, visualize situations that have made you angry in the past—some jerk cut you off on the ramp to the highway, almost causing a collision, or your husband came home from work an hour late without calling—and use progressive muscle relaxation (concentrating on relaxing each major muscle group from your head to your feet) or deep-breathing techniques to quell your anger and calm the tension in your body. By practicing this outside the heat of the moment, the next time your anger is activated, you can use one of these techniques to defuse your reaction quickly. (See "Acting as Your Own Personal Coach," p. 161, for specifics on practicing muscle relaxation.)

Change your thought process.

Psychologists call this cognitive restructuring, and the idea is to tune into the kinds of thoughts that contribute to your anger or cause it to escalate, then to look at them critically, and change the patterns that are counter-productive. For example, if your boss has been giving you extra assignments lately, and that's been making you mad, think about other possible explanations (besides that she's targeting you unfairly). Maybe she's feeling a lot of pressure and she knows she can count on you to help her look good; or maybe she's trying to give you more visibility in the company because she thinks you deserve a promotion. Of course, you could always ask her why she's giving you the extra assignment. Learning to view situations in a more positive or more neutral light can help you nip anger in the bud and take a more constructive approach to resolving the underlying issues.

Try behaving differently.

Instead of squelching your anger, becoming accusatory or eating out your frustrations, face the situation directly. Focus on what's really bothering you, then express yourself in a nonconfrontational way—by describing your thoughts and feelings, using "I" statements rather than hurling accusations. If you practice facing situations that upset you, gradually they'll stop triggering such an intense emotional reaction—or the desire to nosh.

The Power of Self-Talk

If you're really going to change self-limiting patterns of behavior, you're probably going to need to change the way you speak to *yourself.* After all, what you say to yourself is usually an extension of your beliefs. We all talk to ourselves on a regular basis throughout the day, and this commentary typically revolves around the obstacles and opportunities we face. Yet people often don't even realize that their inner voice is speaking; they simply accept what it has to say as the gospel truth. Psychologists call this self-talk, and they have found that what you tell yourself can have a profound effect, for better or worse, on how you feel, what you do, and how you see the world. Depending on the content of these internal messages, they can either help or hinder your performance—and your ability to reach your goals.

Athletes frequently use self-talk as a coping mechanism to help themselves stay calm, cool, collected, and focused when they experience mounting pressure to perform at their peak. And research has found that positive self-talk—having an internal voice that's upbeat, encouraging and constructive—can help people feel more confident and focused in everyday life. It's a way of taking charge of the thoughts and messages that naturally run through your mind as you prepare for a challenge or face it directly. It's also a way of using intentional, logical thought to guide your attitude and your behavior as you strive to accomplish your goals.

Research has found, for example, that self-talk can help people build a self-concept, or an image of themselves, because it helps them make inferences about themselves. It can also help people make savvy choices: When researchers at the University of Louisville examined how often college students engaged in positive self-talk and how often they practiced various health behaviors, it turned out that positive self-talk was highly correlated with students' participation in vigorous exercise, their use of seat belts, and avoiding alcoholic beverages. Another study found that saying more positive things and fewer negative things to themselves than usual helped a group of women achieve a greater level of pain tolerance than normal. Meanwhile, a Canadian study found that positive self-talk strategies helped a group of athletes persevere longer on a muscular leg-endurance task than athletes who were instructed to focus on the challenge or disassociate from it.

By contrast, negative self-talk—being overly critical of yourself, predicting doom or disaster, blaming yourself unfairly for the outcome of a situation or simply saying nasty things to yourself—can be downright detrimental to your well-being. Not only can it make you feel lousy about yourself, but it can also cause creative blocks and anxiety, undermine your confidence, destroy your concentration and ultimately thwart your ability to achieve your goals. It's like having a harsh critic take up residence in your head: Once that happens, you are constantly subjected to the tyranny of negative judgments and emotional abuse. As unpleasant as this sounds, the real problem occurs when you start to believe or accept what that inner critic is saying.

Negative self-talk can become a particularly prickly issue when you're striving to change your ways. We all crave continuity at heart. So when you try to change a habit, internal voices of discouragement will naturally pipe up and protest the shift from the status quo. What you need to do when that happens is recognize that these are the voices of resistance, and refrain from taking their advice. When those discouraging voices chime in, remind yourself why you want to make the change you're striving for and how it will improve your life in the long run. If you want to stop smoking and a little voice inside you says, "Come on, have just one," hold it right there and point out that quitting will help you breathe a lot easier and dramatically lower your risk of developing lung cancer.

Pay attention to what you say to yourself and change it when necessary. Your inner naysayer is simply spewing out information that travels through your belief and thought systems; rather than being based on fact, it usually stems from cognitive distortions, or, in layman's terms, twisted thoughts. Often, these negative thinking patterns come from people's childhood experiences. If you grew up in a household where one of your parents was highly critical of you, for example, you may have internalized these messages, giving birth to your inner critic. But that doesn't mean you have to continue living with her. You can—and should—evict her.

Once you become attuned to the negative or discouraging things you say to yourself, you can replace those misguided thoughts with more positive or constructive messages. If you're truly out of touch with the critic in your head, it might help to jot down the negative things you say to yourself for three consecutive days and make a note of what was going on when the inner critic piped up. If you realize you're calling yourself a complete idiot for some social faux pas you committed, remind yourself that you're *not* a complete idiot, that you simply didn't handle the situation as well as you could have and that you need to be more careful next time.

Or you could take it a step further and use affirmations to buoy your confidence: If you're about to go into a meeting where crucial decisions will be made on the spot, you might tell yourself, "I am a quick thinker and I generally come through under pressure." Consciously making this conversion from the inner naysayer to the positive inner coach helps this more encouraging voice gradually become the louder one.

Acting as Your Own Personal Coach

Being a more positive inner coach needn't mean that you should put a positive spin on everything—that would be like donning rose-colored glasses, which won't help you in your pursuit of excellence *or* your quest for self-improvement. This isn't about the power of positive thinking; it's about the power of effective self-coaching. After all, unless your positive thoughts lead to effective action, those thoughts aren't especially useful.

Instead of bombarding yourself with superficially positive messages, it's more effective to analyze your performance or your preparation constructively in an effort to give yourself effective coaching and the best chance to succeed. To do that, you'll need to be honest about your weaknesses without being overly critical of yourself.

A constructive inner coach can help you do this. By identifying areas you need to work on, your inner coach can help you focus your attention

Deciding How You Measure Up

Nearly everyone does it. And, indeed, psychologists have found that it's hard for people not to compare themselves with others, especially in situations where objective standards aren't available.

But comparing yourself to other people can be risky business. For one thing, it often raises the bar to unattainable standards—trying to be the absolute best among your peers, for example, instead of striving to be the best that you can possibly be. It focuses on the endpoint or the desired result, rather than what you can do to improve yourself or your situation. As a result, comparing yourself to others can divert your attention from what you should be doing to pursue your goals. Worse, playing the social comparison game can needlessly lead to a drop in self-esteem, in some instances.

Interestingly enough, research from the University of Waterloo in Ontario, Canada, found that people prefer to contrast their current status with their past status when they want to feel good—or at least adequate—about themselves; this form of comparison reflects improvement over time, which can be gratifying. But when people want to obtain an accurate assessment of how they're doing, they generally prefer to compare themselves with other people, according to several studies.

In addition, a person's self-esteem may play a role in determining which form of comparison she naturally gravitates to. A study from the University of California at Los Angeles found that people who have high self-esteem generally use personal standards to evaluate how they're doing, whereas those who have low self-esteem more often rely on social comparison.

This natural proclivity for people to compare their current selves with their past selves may not continue throughout adulthood, how-

continued on next page

ever. As people age and some of their physical and cognitive skills decline, it may be *less* discouraging to compare oneself with a group of peers than to the person of one's youth. Indeed, a study from the University of Wisconsin found that while young and middle-aged adults saw considerable improvements in their well-being from the past to the present, older adults were more likely to see themselves as holding steady; moreover, whereas the young and middle-aged adults expected continued gains in the coming years, the older people expected a decline in most aspects of their well-being.

The bottom line: It pays to be careful about how you measure your own progress. If your intention is to sustain motivation, you'd be wise to judge your own personal improvements. If what you want is a reality check, however, it might be better to gauge how you're doing compared to similarly matched peers. But make sure that you compare yourself only to people who have similar characteristics relevant to the issue at hand (skills, intelligence, experience). Otherwise, you're simply being unfair to yourself.

and your efforts on what you need to do to succeed. She can be observant, and can make helpful suggestions without being negative or nasty. Whereas your inner critic might discourage improvement with her negative commentary, your inner coach will encourage positive changes with her supportive style. Let's say you want to make a first-rate presentation to your boss or you want to use your wicked serve to your best advantage in an upcoming tennis match. Right before you're about to act, your inner critic would probably chime in with a reminder about the last presentation you blew or how often you double-faulted the last time you competed in a tournament. Your personal coach will point out that you've been working on these skills, and that you've improved them dramatically. She might tell you that you're much more prepared going into this challenge than you were for the last one and that you've got the right mind-set this time around.

But here's the hitch: You'll need to practice this positive self-talk on a regular basis if you want the more constructive dialogue to eventually come naturally. It can be done, but it probably won't be easy. On the contrary, sometimes it may be difficult to come up with a more constructive alternative to what your inner critic is saying. But you can do it if you employ the following tactics to bolster your performance in a given situation:

* **Forget about the results and focus on your actions.** Remind yourself that you can't control the outcome but you can control your actions, so that's where your attention should be directed. Try to block out thoughts about the result you're aiming for and concentrate, instead, on what you need to do right now to perform at your best.

* **Find the lesson in what goes wrong.** People who succeed in their endeavors often view their mistakes as opportunities for learning. Rather than berate themselves for what they did wrong or simply accept defeat, they examine the situation for possible solutions for the future. They're not afraid to ask questions like "What can I do differently next time to improve my performance?" When handled this way, it's impossible for mistakes to lead to failure because you'll learn from the experience, and that knowledge will help you move toward your goals.

* **Zero in on how you'll handle your weak spots.** Take a look at the course you've charted for yourself as you strive for your goals and identify which particular points might be problematic for you, then come up with a strategy for how you'll navigate your way through that treacherous terrain. For example, it might be a good idea to slow your pace or ask for assistance, if that will ultimately further your progress.

* **Keep rehearsing success in your mind.** By continuously visualizing the event and how you'll act during it, you'll be preparing yourself to do what it takes to turn your dreams into reality. The key is to marshal all your imaginative powers to create the scene—and your behavior in it— exactly as you want it to actually unfold.

* **Put history in its proper place.** Remind yourself that each situation offers a brand-new opportunity to succeed. That means that whatever

happened in similar situations in the past is nothing more than history; it has no bearing on how you'll do in the present. The slate is clean. So buckle down and focus on what you need to do *now*.

◆ **Remember what it is that you do right.** Rather than focus on your mistakes or shortcomings, point out all the qualities you have going for you—your eye for detail, your ability to think on your feet, your enthusiasm—before going to a job interview, for example. Replay past successes in your mind to bolster your confidence.

◆ **Reinforce your mental vigor.** You can use affirmations to your advantage as long as you don't try to falsely brainwash yourself into a positive state of mind. Affirmations won't work their magic if you don't believe them, that's why it's essential to make these self-statements as specific as possible so that they actually correspond to aspects of your preparation and training that you deserve to feel confident about. You might tell yourself, "I've practiced this presentation dozens of times; I'm ready to go" or "I have the physical skills to succeed in this challenge." You can use affirmations to remind yourself that your goal is worth pursuing, that you are capable of achieving it, and that you deserve to succeed.

◆ **Help yourself relax under pressure.** There's nothing wrong with being nervous before a big event. Trouble arises, however, when that nervousness is given the chance to impede or interfere with your performance. That's why the personal coach inside you should encourage you to relax by learning and practicing techniques such as deep breathing, muscle relaxation or visualization. Here are the basics:

With deep breathing, you want to use your diaphragm rather than your chest muscles. Imagine there is a grapefruit located just behind your belly button; inhale slowly and imagine that air is filling up that grapefruit by passing directly through your belly button. Then slowly let the air escape, again through your belly button, as you exhale.

With progressive muscle relaxation, the aim is alternately to tense and then relax each set of muscles from your head to your toes. You might start with your neck and consciously tighten the muscles for three seconds, then fully relax them, imagining them becoming warm and heavy. Progress to your shoulders, then to your chest, your arms and hands, your abdomen, your buttocks, your thighs, your lower legs and, finally, to your feet.

With visualization techniques, you close your eyes and picture a tranquil scene, using all your senses to create a vivid image. If you've chosen to visualize a day at the beach, you might focus on the clear blue of the sky, the smell and taste of the salty air, the feel of a gentle breeze, the soothing sound of the waves lapping up onto the shore, the texture of the sand between your toes. Breathe deeply as you imagine this scene for 10 to 15 minutes, then open your eyes and enjoy your relaxed state.

The key to using each of these techniques effectively is to employ them regularly in everyday life. This is yet another example of how practice makes perfect: By using these skills when you aren't under pressure, you'll be able to rely upon them when you truly need them to help you navigate through a difficult situation.

When you can begin to shed your unrealistic beliefs, silence your inner critic, and amplify your personal coach's voice, you'll be priming the pump for success. Getting rid of *should* and *must* and replacing them with *can* and *will* is both liberating and inspiring because it puts you in charge of both your thoughts and your actions. Plus, by choosing to reframe your beliefs and style of self-talk in a more constructive light, you'll be bolstering your chances to achieve your goals because success will feel more possible, perhaps even likely. Making the switch takes time, practice and patience. But it can be done. Whenever you catch yourself making the conversion, pause for a moment and give yourself a pat on the back, just as a good coach would.

Are You a Good Friend to Yourself?

If you're like many women, you rally to the defense of your friends when someone speaks poorly of them. You tell them they're being too hard on themselves when they're filled with self-blame or self-criticism. And you probably try to bolster their spirits when life throws them a curve ball. Do you provide yourself with the same kindness and care? You can find out by taking this mini quiz.

1. When you run into an acquaintance at the grocery store, she seems a bit chilly. Your reaction is to:
   a) *rack your brain trying to think of what you might have done to offend her.*
   b) *dismiss her behavior as a sign that she's simply having a bad day.*

2. While having lunch with a colleague who has been feeling blue, you start feeling as sad or anxious as she does. You:
   a) *don't think anything of it; moods come and go all the time.*
   b) *realize it's because you're catching her mood and give yourself a quick time-out by excusing yourself for a trip to the ladies' room.*

3. After a presentation you've given at work bombs, you are most likely to:
   a) *go over and over the material, trying to pinpoint where you went wrong.*
   b) *initiate damage control by writing a follow-up memo.*

4. When faced with a vexing decision, you are more likely to:
   a) *take a poll among friends about what you should do or get someone else to make the decision for you.*
   b) *remind yourself that few decisions are irrevocable or unfixable, then make a list of solutions that could possibly work.*

5. Your spouse calls Friday afternoon with bad news: He won't be able to go away for the weekend as you'd planned because he got socked with a last-minute project at work. You:
   a) *can't help but think about how much you needed this getaway, about how hard it is to get time alone with him, about how his job always seems to get in the way of family plans.*
   b) *feel disappointed—who wouldn't?—but try to come up with something fun for you to do by yourself or with a friend instead.*

Tally the number of times you chose a or b. If you scored more a's, you have some emotional bad habits that are preventing you from treating yourself as well as you should—in which case it's time to change your attitude and thought patterns. If you chose more b's, congratulations! You're being as caring and considerate toward yourself as you would be toward a dear friend. And that's the way it should be.

ASSIGNMENT Think about a recent situation where just about everything went wrong in your performance, whether it was during a presentation at work, an athletic event, or a social gathering. Now consider how your thought patterns may have contributed to the downward spiral. How did you assess the situation? What kinds of things did you say to yourself about your appearance or behavior? Next, while imagining the circumstances as vividly as possible, think about what you could have said to yourself that would have been more constructive and helpful. How could you have helped yourself concentrate more effectively? How could you have improved the way you presented yourself or the way you made decisions? By reviewing this situation and brainstorming about what you could have done differently, you'll help prepare your inner coach—and silence your inner critic—for the next challenge that lies ahead.

CHAPTER EIGHT

Try the Flip Side

There's a piece of Weight Watchers wisdom that really embraces the spirit of change: "If you keep doing what you've always done then you'll always get what you've always gotten." What sounds so simple in fact eludes most of us. It can be exceedingly difficult to change ingrained habits and, as anyone with a weight problem can attest, changing our eating habits can seem almost impossible. All the negativity we attach to dieting doesn't help either. Conventional thinking about starving ourselves thin is enough to doom anyone to dieting failure. But what would happen if we flipped that notion around and said you can eat more and still lose weight? We'd be drawn to the prospect, wouldn't we? There was a time when the bane of my overweight life was that I felt like a failure until I could fit into a skinny dress. I felt deprived when I starved myself and guilty when I ate out of frustration. I always felt self-conscious when I exercised, even more so about getting into a swimsuit, riding jodhpurs or a tennis shift, even though I excelled at sports. It's no wonder I loathed dieting and myself along with it. It was not until I joined Weight Watchers that I gave up myths steeped in negativity and discovered that dieting can be an amazing journey where we gradually choose to give up old habits for far better ones.

In this chapter you'll see how Weight Watchers leader Michelle Seymour released herself from a maddening cycle of gaining and losing weight and in the process unlocked the secret to keeping it off. Michelle used to be so focused on reaching her goal weight that she would do whatever she

How to Take a Vacation from Your Worries

When setbacks occur or you begin to feel stuck in your life, there's often a natural tendency to go over and over a vexing situation in your mind, in the hope that you'll have a "Eureka!" moment and seize upon the solution. Unfortunately, it doesn't usually happen that way. The reality is, this approach, which psychologists call rumination, can be *counter*productive. It's a case where too much analysis can lead to paralysis, preventing you from doing something about what's troubling you.

Research has found that rumination is more common among women, notes Susan Nolen-Hoeksema, Ph.D., an associate professor of psychology at the University of Michigan, and it may partly explain why women are twice as prone to depression as men are. "When people ruminate," she explains, "there's a spiraling downward into a deeper and deeper hole, which tends to make them feel worse and makes it harder to take positive action." They spend much of their time dwelling on how bad they feel, as well as on the consequences of their emotions. And they continue doing this over and over again without taking action to move forward or to use more positive coping strategies.

A better approach: Distract yourself from the problem or your feelings for a while—by exercising, engaging in a hobby or talking to a trusted friend—and set worry hours for later, whether it's later that day or week. Choose a time when you can go back and address the problem with a fresh point of view. At that point, it can help to brainstorm by writing down your concerns along with potential solutions. It's also a good idea to use friends as sounding boards; ask them to give you a reality check on when your concerns seem realistic (or not) and how you might deal more effectively with them. If it turns out that you can't exert any influence over the problem at hand, you'd be better off accepting that, trying to learn from the experience and turning your attention to matters you can do something about.

had to do to achieve it. She'd skip breakfast not realizing that later on she'd overeat out of hunger. As a busy mother of young children, Michelle's attempts at exercise were too sporadic to make a difference. Looking back, Michelle can see that efforts to slim down were short-lived at best mainly because she treated change as a series of isolated tasks rather than integrating them into a new and healthier lifestyle. She started to see things differently after she began attending Weight Watchers meetings. She says the meetings opened her mind to the wisdom and experience of others who were succeeding at losing weight on the program. Instead of sounding war weary, these dieters were full of joy and enthusiasm—and most had not even reached their goal yet!

Where is it written that you don't succeed on a diet until you reach your weight goal? A more motivating approach says that *any* weight loss qualifies as success and that a succession of interim victories can help sustain our motivation when our goal seems far off. When we are motivated by success instead of the fear of failure, our mind and body lead us to believe in our ability to achieve our goals. I especially like what Michelle says about our power of choice as far as adopting a winning attitude is concerned. Imagine the universe is neutral, she says, and whether it is a positive or negative place depends on how we choose to experience it. Michelle said she became a winner at weight loss when she started to see herself as a winner. Even when Michelle gained 10 pounds after the death of her mother, she called herself a learner, not a failure. I too gained weight after my own mother's death, and the truth is that giving some power back to food was part of my grieving and healing process. It made me stronger because I had the tools and confidence I needed to get back on track when I was emotionally ready. I agree that everyone is different and that there's no one answer to everyone's weight problems. We are all unique and each of us knows deep down what's right and what's not right in our life.

Michelle acknowledges that the majority of people who struggle with weight have an innate sense of what they want, but she finds that their weakened self-esteem can make change difficult. At some point some people cannot ignore that sense of truth in themselves, and they finally act on their desire for change. It is at this moment that the opportunity to start building self-esteem kicks in, because each new round of challenge and accomplishment can be very empowering. Consider that nowhere in our vocabulary will you find the term "other-people-esteem." We call it "self-esteem" because it's a feeling we cultivate in ourselves largely by ourselves based on what we know is right and true to our heart. It's never too late to start, because as with losing weight, we all take it one step at a time.

Profile: Michelle Seymour
Learning to Do Things Differently

Michelle Seymour was always thin as a kid, and she maintained a normal weight during her teenage and college years. Of course, like many women, she would gain five pounds every now and then—around the holidays, for example—but they always came off without much of a battle. "My mother was always a struggling Weight Watchers member, and all of the women in my family have, sooner or later, had weight issues," says Seymour, now 41 and a mother of five in New Jersey. Michelle had a feeling that she, too, would eventually follow in their footsteps.

And indeed she did, after she got married, had two kids, and turned 30. Suddenly, she had 35 pounds to lose from her 5-foot 8-inch frame. "I'd had two babies in 18 months, and I was wearing only maternity clothes because I wasn't able to fit into my other clothes," she recalls. "I only gained weight from my underwear down— behind a desk I looked fine, but not as I left the room. It got to the point where I had two skirts with elastic waists and one pair of jeans. That's all I wore for a year."

In 1989, in the midst of planning a trip to the beach, Michelle decided to join Weight Watchers with her sister-in-law. She lost the weight easily enough, but within six months she'd regained half of it. In 1990, she joined Weight Watchers again and lost the weight for good. She's been a Weight Watchers leader ever since.

The biggest obstacle to losing the weight and keeping it off lay in her mind-set, she says. "The first time I lost weight, I was so goal-oriented," she explains. "I treated it like a diet, and I had the belief that if you dieted your weight off, it was off and you'd never have to worry about it again—you'd be finished. When I gained the weight back, I realized I had to change my approach because I was setting myself up to fail instead of succeed. I realized there had to be absolute consistency in what I was trying to do. Our bodies are going to follow natural law—whatever you do repeatedly, your body will show. Weddings and holidays are not everyday events; you go to them—and maybe you eat too much—but then you go back to what you do every day."

Realizing this, and attending the Weight Watchers' meetings, gave Michelle the senses of accountability and responsibility she needed to slim down once and for all. "It was so important to me not to regain the weight that I was willing to toss aside my beliefs and try the ideas from people in the meetings," she recalls. "I had to listen to people who were successful and implement some of their ideas."

How did she shake up her routine and revamp her lifestyle habits? "I began to get rid of mindless eating and I realized that exercise had to become a part of how I conducted business," Michelle explains. "And I found lower-calorie and lower-fat options. I used to put butter, cheese or mayonnaise on just about everything. I started using marinades for meat, low-fat or fat-free salad dressings and more spices and herbs. And I had to learn that calories were calories but it was important to feed your body on a consistent schedule." Michelle used to be a breakfast skipper but she started forcing herself to eat a morning meal, which made her less of a nighttime nosher. "I've found that if I eat breakfast and lunch, it's easier for me to eat a healthy dinner than if I were extremely hungry from skipping meals," she says. "And I started allowing myself to eat treats as they were designed to be eaten—as treats—rather than as a meal."

With the help of other Weight Watchers members, she began to look at slip-ups in a different light, too: "I used to have the idea that if I had a cookie my day was ruined because I broke my diet," Michelle explains. "So I figured I might as well go to the freezer with a spoon and no bowl and have all the ice cream I wanted. Another lesson I learned is that any time I make an error, it's not a failure; it's just an error and there's something to be learned from it. That ability to pick myself up after a slip, rather than lie down and wait for a truck to roll over me, is possibly the greatest thing I got from Weight Watchers."

Indeed, changing her eating habits gave Michelle a new vision of what it takes to lead a healthy lifestyle. And as she lost weight, she gained a new perspective of herself, too. "It strengthened my belief that I could do what I set out to do and it changed my belief that all of the women in my family have to be heavy," she says. "The experience has taught me to take the necessary small steps to get from where I am to where I want to be. I don't look at any task as too daunting or too large. I just start and take the first step, then I decide what the next step is going to be."

But Michelle has also learned to keep the big picture in mind—when it comes to maintaining her slim shape as well as in other areas of her life, such as child-rearing. And that's why she went to work for Weight Watchers and now leads 13 meetings a week. "I got hooked on seeing the elevation of the human spirit that comes from losing weight, on watching people absolutely change their lives because they've changed the size of their bodies," she explains. "It's so empowering to watch people take control of their lives by taking control of their eating habits and by exercising. It's an internal drive. It's not that their hips are suddenly smaller but that they chose to make them smaller. You see it in their eyes when they 'get it.'

"I remember when I got it: I thought I was going to be another overweight, middle-aged mother," recalls Michelle. "But I'm not. Yes, I'm middle-aged, and, yes, I'm a mother. But I've changed my definition of myself. I had always had a singular definition of myself—as a student or as a wife—and I realized it didn't have to be that way. I'm a working woman who has a family, and I like that I'm a good role model for my children. I now consider myself stronger and more in control in every area of my life. I feel like anything I undertake I can accomplish because losing weight and keeping it off taught me that I have that ability."

BY PURSUING THE GOALS you've set for yourself, you've already pushed yourself to get out of your comfort zone and explore personally uncharted territory. By simply adopting new behaviors you've already scored a victory for yourself because it has undoubtedly led to self-growth. But in the process of change, there often comes a time when the tried-and-true strategies you've been relying on suddenly seem to let you down. When progress is no longer going according to plan—if you reach a plateau in your weight-loss efforts, for instance, or your once budding career seems to have stalled out—you can begin to feel depleted of the personal energy and resources that it takes to continue striving for your goals.

Believe it or not, this is a common phenomenon—and it may stem, in large part, from the stress and sustained attention that are involved in trying to continually control yourself. Indeed, research has found that trying to regulate yourself intensely can make you downright tired. In one study, researchers at Case Western Reserve University in Cleveland, Ohio, found that when people tried to regulate their emotional response to an upsetting movie, they subsequently experienced a decrease in physical stamina. Moreover, a study from the University of Cincinnati found that having to pay sustained attention to something led to fidgeting and fatigue. So there really is a psychological and physiological basis for running out of gas in the midst of an intense pursuit.

It's important to remember that temporary setbacks like this are normal. Life has peaks and valleys, and these can affect your performance. But that doesn't mean you should give up when things aren't going your way. It simply means that you should start handling them differently. You don't necessarily have to work harder; it may simply be a matter of working smarter or trying a strategy that you wouldn't ordinarily consider. In fact, if you really feel as though your progress has slowed or as though the spark of your motivation is flickering, it's a mistake to keep pushing ahead using the same strategies. Persistence and self-discipline are noble attributes, but it's important to know when to back off or when to rewrite the rules. Otherwise, you could wind up courting burnout: physical, emotional and mental exhaustion. Psychologists say the potential for burnout increases dramatically if you're a diligent worker who constantly gives 110 percent or if you're an idealistic, self-motivated achiever who continues to believe that anything is possible if you continue to work long enough and hard enough.

Indeed, sometimes it's better to shake up your routine rather than to simply proceed with business as usual or push yourself even harder. The key is to dare to do things differently, because what you're doing now is no longer as effective as it was. Believe it or not, this is yet another way in which the process of change requires you to venture out of your comfort zone. Even the pursuit of a particular goal can take place within your comfort zone if you go about it the same way day after day. But since you're striving for self-improvement, you might think it's okay to be in this comfort zone. Why should you bother to leave what's comfortable and familiar since you're already under pressure to perform well? The answer is that in the end, being too comfortable can hold you back from continuing to evolve and make progress toward your goals.

Even if you have already achieved some degree of change in your life, going further is still up to you. And each time you strive for something new—even if it's simply a different way of pursuing the same goals—you step out of your comfort zone. It could be a giant step or a baby step, but it takes you out of the cozy territory of complacency. In the process of pursuing a new challenge and gaining confidence in yourself, your comfort zone has probably already expanded considerably. But living inside the confines of your comfort zone can be detrimental to your personal growth and well-being. When you are exposed to patterns of people and situations that are perceived as "the same old, same old," you may unconsciously "shut down" because you are not receiving any new stimulation, according to Ellen J. Langer, Ph.D., a professor of psychology at Harvard University. And that can put you right back where you don't want to be—on automatic pilot.

Sneaky Situations That Can Snare Your Progress

The road to changing your life is paved with potholes and roadblocks. If you avert your attention and let down your guard, your pursuit of your goals can take a sharp, unwanted detour. But if you keep your eyes on the road ahead, you can often steer clear of such glitches or at least navigate your way through them safely. Here are four commonly encountered situations that can thwart your efforts in various aspects of your life, along with strategies on how to deal with them:

Situation: Your weight loss has plateaued and you're feeling incredibly frustrated.

Solution: First, rest assured this is a common problem. Nearly every person who has ever tried to lose a substantial amount of weight has hit a plateau and has felt the aggravation you're now experiencing. Plateaus can happen for a number of reasons. It may be that your body just needs a break from all the changes it has weathered. Or it could be that you've returned to some of your old eating habits without realizing it. That's why it's a good idea to take a close look at your eating and exercise patterns to make sure that you're truly sticking with your plan. If you really are, try to relax, continue with your current dietary regimen and stay physically active. Chances are, once your body adjusts to your new, lower weight, you'll begin to peel off pounds again.

Situation: Your boss reassigns a prized project or client to someone else.

Solution: There's no question that this would be a tremendous disappointment, and you'd probably read quite a bit of negative stuff between the lines. You might even feel humiliated. Try to put aside your feelings for the moment, and focus on what might have gone wrong and what you could try to do to remedy the situation. When you feel up to it, schedule a meeting with your boss and try to find out where you need to improve and what projects you can take on that will enhance these skills. By having this frank discussion, you might learn that the reassignment actually had nothing to do with you, that it was a political move within the company (maybe another department head wants to oversee that project). But even if the change was related to your performance, you'll know what you need to do to improve for the future.

Situation: You're working out longer and harder but you're getting less out of exercise.

Solution: It may be that the law of diminishing returns has kicked in. Often, people who jump on the exercise bandwagon push themselves too far, too fast. While it may seem as though working out every day is a great way to get in shape quickly, it can set you up for injuries or physical burnout. After exercise, the body needs time to replenish its energy stores and repair muscles. So if you're getting less and less out of your workouts, you may want to get in the habit of exercising every other day or alternating intense workouts with lighter ones such as gentle walking. It's all a matter of balance.

Situation: You've put yourself on a strict budget but you don't seem to be saving much money.

Solution: It could be that you've slashed major expenditures but you're neglecting some of the details of your spending habits—like the daily latte you treat yourself to or the magazine you regularly buy for your train ride home. These little items add up over time. To get to the bottom of your spending habits, put away your credit cards and start using cold, hard cash for all your purchases. Next, start writing down all your expenditures—the big ones and the little ones—for a month or two to get a clear sense of your spending habits. Compare your expenditures to the amount of money you have coming in each month, and, if you need to, figure out how you can cut costs a little more—by buying store brands instead of national brands, or by borrowing books from the library instead of buying your own, for example. This can help you reach your savings goals.

Getting Unstuck

Whether it's your weight, your job or a relationship, if you feel as though you're at a standstill, you might be wondering what went wrong. It may be that complacency or stagnation has taken up residence in your attitude without your realizing it. It may be that you are now simply going through the motions of pursuing your goals without daring to take chances, try new techniques or venture into unknown arenas. Or it may be that you're being too hard on yourself, that you've been holding yourself to standards that are too high. In fact, a study from St. Bartholomew's Hospital in London found that perfectionism is a serious factor in the development of long-term unexplained fatigue.

Regardless of what has caused you to feel as though you're treading water, what you want to do at this point is to envision new ways to tackle your challenges. You'll need to find a detour or an alternate route around whatever obstacle is standing in your way that will still deliver you to your chosen destination. Granted, it's not easy to shed past approaches, especially if they've worked for you before. Often that's because people are particularly reluctant to let go of previous strategies out of fear that they'll need to learn new skills or acquire more knowledge to continue making progress on their goals. But that's not always true. It may be that something in your current approach is holding you back, in which case letting go of the problematic aspect may be enough to initiate forward progress. In other instances, sometimes it's a matter of trying something completely different or simply applying skills you've employed in other areas of your life to the challenge at hand.

For example, it could be that your career progress has been stymied because of the way you handle criticism—namely, by reacting defensively instead of trying to learn from it; in that case, letting go of this approach by making an effort to take supervisors' comments to heart and trying to improve your performance based on what they've said could be all you need to do to earn that coveted promotion. It could be that you've been subtly compromising your weight-loss efforts by skipping breakfast on a daily basis, which sets you up for overeating the rest of the day; by making the switch to eating a morning meal, you might find that you can keep your appetite under better control all day long.

In both instances, you need to get out of your own way. In order to do that, you'll need to uncover the hidden psychological roadblocks that may be impeding your progress. Keep your eyes on the goal but don't be afraid to experiment, to play against the grain, to rewrite the rules you've set for yourself; in other words, be willing to be flexible and do the opposite of what comes naturally. Achieving your goals requires that you have the *will* and the *way*, and if the old way isn't working, it's time to cultivate a new one. Here are fourteen ways to get out of a behavioral rut:

Find the automatic pilot controls. It could be that you've started relying on one set of rules or strategies. When you continue to use the same tactics even when they are no longer working for you, that constitutes automatic or mindless behavior. Becoming aware of this pattern might inspire you to create new guidelines or strategies. If you've been using the same boilerplate format for your reports at work, for example, and they're no longer garnering the attention and praise that they once did, you may need to discover or develop a new style for presenting your ideas. If your daily two-mile walk no longer seems to be doing the trick, perhaps you need to up your mileage, walk in a new location or change your workout altogether.

Try to see life from more than one angle. It's not just a question of being open to new information and novel strategies, it's also important to appreciate different points of view. Not only will this help you gain insight into different approaches that might work, but it can also help you recognize other options for responding to a particular situation and help you develop empathy, which can enhance your relationships with other people. If you and your spouse have been butting heads again and again over your respective ideas about managing your finances, for example, try to see matters from his point of view: Maybe you'll realize that his approach has roots in psychological insecurities about money that stem from his family of origin. Seeing things from another angle can help take the heat out of a conflict, but it can also help you identify other solutions—or compromises—to deal with conflicts.

Expose yourself to the right kind of stimulation. Too little external stimulation in everyday life can be as harmful as too much. In fact, research has found that *both* can lead to profound fatigue. In a study conducted at Maastricht University in the Netherlands, researchers discovered that an overload of stimulation and low-quality stimulation were both linked with higher reports of fatigue among 777 participants. You want to aim for a balance between the amount of sensory and intellectual stimulation you receive—enough to keep you engaged and interested but not so much that you feel overwhelmed. In addition, you want to try to weed out as much of the low-quality or less attractive stimulation—such as noise, excessively bright lights, offending scents—as possible.

Turn a stumbling block into a stepping-stone. When you suffer a setback—whether it's gaining a few pounds or getting a job transfer that isn't a promotion—pick yourself up and try to learn from what happened. If a tactic you tried didn't lead to the results you'd hoped for, it's time to try another approach. Try to find a way to reposition yourself and use this change to your advantage. Maybe you can tinker with the content of your diet so that it helps you feel more satiated and less prone to snacking. Maybe you can use some of the skills you honed at your old job to make yourself indispensable in your new department or office. When viewed in this light, there's no such thing as failure because every experience, even one that goes awry, becomes an opportunity for learning.

Give your beliefs a checkup. First examine the form of behavior

Making Emotional Changes

Sometimes it can take a while for your emotions to catch up to the physical, behavorial or circumstantial changes you've made in your life. When that happens, you might feel uneasy acting in your new style or you might even feel uncomfortable in your own skin if your appearance has changed considerably. While you're grappling with these feelings of discomfort, reverting to your old ways can seem exceedingly appealing.

Don't do it. Eventually your comfort quotient will catch up with the changes you've made. In the meantime, the key is to try to tolerate these ambivalent feelings as best you can—and to realize they're nothing more than a phase that will pass. Acknowledging your feelings of discomfort (to yourself) is a step in the right direction; by naming the feeling and where it comes from, it may seem less unsettling to you. It also may help to probe the feeling a bit, in order to reveal its underpinnings.

How to do this: Describe this feeling of uneasiness using as many different adjectives or phrases as you need to accurately capture it. Next, consider how this feeling affects your actions, your thoughts and your life. And finally, think about what you could do now to defuse the feeling, rechannel it or move through it. For example, if you're feeling uncomfortable with your newly slim shape, rather than overeating, try to discover what's really making you feel uncomfortable. Is it all the extra energy you have (which could be making you feel wired or anxious) or the fact that you're getting more physical attention than you used to? Then, when you consider how you can prevent these feelings from having a negative impact on your life, you might realize that exercising more vigorously could help you burn off that extra energy and make you feel more grounded. As far as being noticed goes, this might be an instance where it

continued on next page

would help to learn to tolerate the feeling—by breathing deeply and trying to relax when you feel uncomfortable or by using the power of positive self-talk to get you through those anxious moments.

Remember: This emotional layover is temporary. As the American inventor Thomas Edison once noted, "Restlessness and discontent are the necessities of progress." You may be able to speed up the dissolution of these feelings by relying on the emotional resources you've been building throughout the process of change. Once again, this will make you your own very best ally—and that can help you feel like you can handle almost anything.

that isn't producing the results you want. Then look at the beliefs that may be driving that behavior. Now consider how you could change those beliefs in such a way that they would likely lead to better results. Maybe you've stopped volunteering for extra projects at work because the last one didn't turn out well, or maybe you've stopped coming to the net on the tennis court because your volleys haven't been up to par. If you really did some soul-searching about your behavior, you might discover that it's because you're afraid of failing again. Perhaps your underlying belief is that failure is bad.

You might then replace that belief with the conviction that what counts is that you try your hardest and that there's nothing wrong with failing as long as you learn from the process. With those beliefs guiding your behavior, you'll be more likely to try new strategies, take smart risks, exercise your talents and expand your horizons—all of which will probably help you improve your performance and your progress toward your goals.

Write a farewell letter. If you suspect that one of your self-limiting beliefs is still impeding your progress, it's time to bid it a formal good-bye in a letter. Address the letter to yourself, and write something along these lines: "I realize *that people wouldn't like me if they knew the real me* [or whatever your self-defeating belief is], but I have decided to move forward with my life so I'll have to let you go. You've served a purpose in my life until now. From this point on, however, I won't be needing you anymore. So it's time for us to say good-bye." Be sure to sign it—in ink. Composing this letter and signing it is a symbolic act that speaks volumes about your intentions to truly and finally let this belief go for good. The result can be invigorating.

Shake it up, baby. When you're stuck in a progress rut, sometimes it helps to shift gears and try doing things differently. This might involve substituting a fresh activity for your usual one (swapping a vigorous bike ride for your jog, for example). It could involve doing your routine at a different time of day (writing your memos in the morning instead of the late afternoon). It might revolve around varying the pace with which you approach your goals (alternating bouts of faster running with slower jogging, for example—what's called interval training). Or you might do what you normally do but in a slightly different form (talking about important matters with your spouse while you cook instead of sitting down for a serious heart-to-heart, for example; or listening to soothing music while you work at your pressure-packed job). The idea is to do something out of the ordinary. Variety isn't just the spice of life; it's a necessary ingredient for keeping your life fresh.

Take a detour and enjoy the sights. If you get off the highway and take a road less traveled toward your desired destination, you might not get there as quickly but you'll observe things you'd otherwise miss, and that could make the experience that much richer. Instead of traveling once again on the well-worn paths of your life, take an alternate route now and then. Not only will this help keep you alert but research has found that it enhances brain function, too. In essence, the new sights, sounds and smells along the way will stimulate the areas of your brain where memory is processed and stored.

Work with your energy cycles. Many people think that energy—physical, emotional, mental and even spiritual energy—should be a constant in their lives. It's not. On the contrary, energy ebbs and flows according to daily, monthly and seasonal rhythms. If you typically feel more energetic over the weekend, it probably means that you're getting a little more sleep and experiencing less stress than during the week. In addition, many women experience bursts of energy just before they get their periods each month. Meanwhile, people who live in northern climates often have lower energy during the winter months, and the arrival of spring and fall tend to bring a renewed sense of vitality.

So, to a certain extent, energy's natural ups and downs are beyond your control. And that means that you shouldn't beat yourself up about low-energy periods in your life. But it also means that you should try to make the most of your natural energy peaks by planning your life—especially the tasks that are involved in pursuing your goals—accordingly.

Let the small stuff go. When you feel that your progress has stalled, it's time to pare down to the essential tasks. Do what's important and be willing to let some things go—or, better yet, delegate them to someone else. It may be that you're suffering from mental weariness, or that you're in danger of burning out on the constant drive for self-improvement. If ever there were a time to give yourself a bit of a break, this is it.

Shift your focus. It's hard to pay attention to the same signals all the time—people talking at a meeting, the news on television, traffic signals and other drivers, and all the other usual stimulus from everyday life. That's why it's smart to focus on another layer of information from time to time. During an extensive business meeting, take a short break and pay attention to the rhythm of your breathing for a few minutes. Or make an effort to really listen to background sounds—the din from the street, the hum of the heater, or whatever it might be. By resting the part of you that you usually use and relying, instead, on another ability or sense, you'll help renew your energy.

Get a life and quit going to extremes. It may be that you're putting too much pressure on yourself to succeed at the expense of other areas of your life. If you've been focusing all your time, energy and attention on trying to earn a promotion, keep doing what you've been doing but pay more attention to your life outside of work—by going to cultural events, getting together with friends more often or participating in enjoyable recreational activities. Similarly, if you've been diligently working to lose weight for months and the possibility of achieving your goal weight has been foremost on your mind, keep up the healthy eating and exercise habits you've cultivated but start thinking about other things as well. Plan a vacation, imagine redecorating your home, read up on current events, volunteer for a community project. Having a fulfilling life and striving passionately for your goals don't have to be mutually exclusive. Besides, living a balanced life has a better chance of helping you attain success with staying power.

Look for the laugh track. One of the most powerful stress relievers around is often overlooked and yet it's free, readily available and doesn't require any skills. It's laughter. Numerous studies have found that laughter and humor can have positive effects such as reducing stress and enhancing immune function. What's more, a sense of humor can boost your ability to bounce back from setbacks. By poking fun at a situation, humor can help you turn reality inside out and upside-down, and that can help you hit upon creative solutions to what's bogging you down at the moment.

Seek advice from those you admire. It's probably time to turn to the role models you identified way back when you were starting this endeavor, or the Board of Advisers you've more recently appointed. Why? Because you could learn from them. They may be able to share some tricks and tactics that worked for them and that could work for you, too. Don't wait for them to deliver their words of wisdom. Take the initiative and contact them; ask them pointed questions about what they did to stay on the path to self-change when they reached a point where the old strategies no longer worked. Ask them if they've noticed any ways in which you might be thwarting your own progress. In all likelihood, they'll be able to locate the wrinkle in what you're doing or offer valuable insights into what worked for them.

By BEING WILLING to do things differently, you'll probably push yourself over the hurdles that have stood in your way. Chances are, you'll also gain a renewed sense of energy and enthusiasm for your mission. That doesn't mean you should count on the rest of the way to be absolutely smooth sailing, however. As the Nobel prize–winning French chemist Marie Curie once noted, "I was taught that the way of progress is neither swift nor easy." Indeed, if it were, achieving your goals wouldn't feel nearly as satisfying.

ASSIGNMENT Outline the major strategies you've been relying upon to lose weight, to land a coveted job or to attain whatever goal you've been striving for. Then, try to come up with a list of five different things you could possibly do to accomplish what you've set your sights on. It might be a matter of trying the opposite approach in some instances. Or it could involve changing your mind-set to take some of the pressure off yourself. Or it might be a matter of setting up your environment or your schedule another way to make your actions feel original. Try to be as specific as possible about what you could dare to do differently. The odds are, this will help you inject a fresh dose of effectiveness and enthusiasm into your pursuit.

CHAPTER NINE

Keep Reaching for the Brass Ring

sometimes have this silly image of my life as a carousel ride with me spinning ever faster around and around. There I am saddled up amid this swirling blur of a dozen painted horses, singing along to the deafening pitch of the pipe organ. My sight is set squarely on the glimmering ring tucked just out of my reach, but with every revolution I lean out farther and farther still—farther in fact than I'd ever imagine possible. I say to myself "Believe and you can have it."

I think everyone's life is like a carousel ride, full of chaotic sights and sounds and the perpetual draw of that brass ring—coveted but dangling just out of arm's reach. Those who remain focused and persistent eventually grab the prize. Some, for all their ups and downs, never do.

I've grabbed the brass ring before and I can tell you that it's worth reaching for. I met and married a wonderful man and together we brought two precious girls into the world. Once I rode nearly 20 hours on horseback across the desert to finish a grueling endurance race. Even the career I enjoy today was unthinkable to me not so long ago. How different my life would be had I never reached for the brass ring and gone beyond what I thought were my own limits.

My friend Maggie Jerchau is a Weight Watchers leader in the New York area, and her experience in overcoming a difficult weight problem is the basis for the chapter you are about to read. She spent years plodding through life feeling terrible about herself and taking on the role of the victim. It's hard for me to imagine Maggie as passive and frustrated because the woman I know is warm, outgoing and very confident.

What was the catalyst to Maggie's transformation? She told me that it began when she'd reached a fork in the road where her options were few and clear: One road would allow her to accept her weight and cope with the consequences it would have on her job and marriage. The other road was no less rocky but it meant digging in and making lasting changes that could lead her to a happier and healthier life.

It was a frightening time in Maggie's life. When confidence is shaky to begin with, we cling to what we know for fear that changes could make things even worse. Fed up with her weight and her life, Maggie set out on a journey of self-discovery that brought surprises at every turn. She joined Weight Watchers and began to talk more openly about her goals and dreams. She started to track her meals and keep a journal. She wasn't an exercise buff but she was able to make walking part of her daily routine.

One change led to another and the signs of progress were clear as she shed more than 70 pounds in less than a year. During that time Maggie came to know what she wanted and acquired the tools to make it all happen. Her new sense of confidence meant she expected more of herself but she also expected more of others, too. As she made her needs clearer to everyone around her, Maggie came to realize that she had the power to shape her world. I can see her now, whirling on her own carousel with her arm outstretched to grasp the brass ring. She didn't get it at first try, but she finally did reach it.

Profile: MAGGIE JERCHAU
Learning to Use My Success as Fuel for the Future

Like many people who wage a war with their weight, Maggie Jerchau had a long history of being overweight, one that dates back to childhood. At age 13, she tipped the scales at close to 190 pounds, but it wasn't until she became interested in boys that she began to think about losing weight. "I tried a million fad diets all through my teens and twenties," admits Maggie, 40, a former nurse who is now a Weight Watchers leader and trainer in New York. During these years, the scale went up and down—and up and down some more. "I could never really keep the weight off," she says. Though she lost weight for her wedding, she gained 10 pounds during her honeymoon, more when they returned home, and retained even more weight after giving birth to her first child, a son.

"As an overweight kid, I tried to fill the needs of other people to gain acceptance," she recalls. "And that's part of the reason I became a nurse—I wanted to be needed, to take care of other people." But while Maggie was tending to other people's needs, she was neglecting her own, a factor that had a profound impact on both her weight history and her inability to lose weight successfully early on. Finally, Maggie became absolutely fed up with her weight struggles in general, and dieting in particular. "At one point, I said to my husband, 'I'm not going to fight this anymore. If I have to be fat for the rest of my life, so be it. And if you can't live with that, you can leave me,'" she recalls. "I was shocked when he said, 'Thank you.' He was so tired of seeing me struggle. He just wanted me to be happy."

While pregnant for the second time, Maggie miscarried during the fifth month of her pregnancy. It was a devastating loss that proved to be the beginning of a turning point for her. "When I lost that baby, that scared me because all my life all I really wanted was to get married and have kids," she explains. "I have an incompetent cervix and at some point somebody asked me if I thought I lost that baby because I was fat. That made me feel so bad, like I had something to do with it, even though my doctor assured me that my weight didn't play a role." Nevertheless, when Maggie became pregnant again three months later and had to be on bedrest for nine months, she changed her approach to eating. "Because I couldn't take control over other areas of my life, I started taking control of what I ate," she explains. "I started eating more healthfully, and, because I was overweight when I became pregnant, I gained only eight pounds during the pregnancy."

Two weeks after giving birth to a healthy baby girl, Maggie went to Weight Watchers with a friend. It was 1988 when she dropped 72½ pounds from her 5-foot 2-inch figure in 10 months. She has kept it off ever since. "I'm very goal-oriented, very determined," she says. "Before this, I had always treated weight issues as a science. And what I realized is I had a lot of emotional challenges to deal with. Food has always been my anesthetic, what I reach for when I need comfort. I needed to develop a different relationship with food."

How did she do that? For starters, she revamped her eating habits: Instead of snacking all day long, as she used to, Maggie began eating three meals a day—including breakfast, which she used to skip—with snacks in between. She became mindful of what she was eating by keeping a food journal. "I had always thought that I didn't eat much but I discovered that I was only counting things I ate when I was sitting down," she says. And she learned to stop blaming external forces—people, situations, and events—for the state of her weight. "I had to take responsibility. I weighed this much because of the choices I made and I had to start making new choices."

Maggie knew that increasing her physical activity would facilitate the weight-loss process, but she'd never been a gym-goer or exercise devotee. "For me, exercise has to be something I fit in step-by-step during the day," she explains. "I take walks when I can, and I park farther away in a lot. I wear a pedometer all day—even when I'm working—so I know if I'm getting enough mileage. When I started doing this, I was doing about a mile per day. Now, on a slow day, I do three miles and often up to eight on a busy day."

As Maggie began developing a healthier lifestyle, she also cultivated other ways of handling herself in situations that were once troubling to her. She needed to figure out how to tap into her inner resources, especially in the face of stress and conflict. "When I was hurting, I started talking or writing about it," she recalls. "I had to face it. In the past, I'd never let myself feel certain emotions, like anger, but I learned to sit with it. Once you learn to let yourself feel emotions, you realize they're not something to fear; they're something that passes just by acknowledgment."

In addition, she needed to find new ways to bolster her confidence and willingness to take a stand on issues she feels are important, rather than squelching her desire to speak up. She did this primarily by learning to talk positively to herself, giving herself pep talks about why she shouldn't sit back and let other people dictate what would happen. She also made a conscious effort to tell other people what she needed and stopped worrying as much about whether others would be upset if they didn't want her to want what she needed. "It still takes a lot of courage for me to stand up and say 'This is what I want,' but it's important for me to do it," she says. "To me, success is the maintenance part of weight loss because in the long run the number doesn't matter. It's the behavior, the relationship you have with food and with yourself that matters. As soon as my eating habits start to change, I know I need to address something within myself. Maintaining my weight means that I'm managing my life and that I'm still an important person in my life. I think I spent most of my life in the victim role—I kind of took what came my way and accepted it. It's a lesson I constantly have to remind myself of even after 12 years—that I have to take care of myself and keep myself a priority; and that in taking care of myself, I'm not taking away from others."

By forcing herself to do this, and by being willing to stand up to new challenges, Maggie gradually became more confident. "I developed a belief in who I was and what I was capable of," she recalls. "I can do this; I can handle this became my credo. I'm stronger—emotionally, physically, psychologically and spiritually—and I'm at peace. That's not to say that peace doesn't get challenged once in a while. But I do have a sense of inner peace and strength. It's self-assurance and confidence that glows from the inside. It affects everything. That sense of self-esteem encouraged me to take on challenges I might not have otherwise, and it's made me a better parent.

"There were a couple of times in my son's grammar school years where my son wasn't being challenged in school because he was so bright," she recalls. "So I made an appointment to discuss this with the principal. It took every ounce of everything I was because it went against everything I was taught as a child. I grew up in an environment where you never questioned or challenged authority. But I learned two things from that experience—that when something is really important to me, it's worth speaking out for. And, second, I earned respect from that principal because I was a parent who believed in her child and was willing to risk her comfort for that belief." Since then, she has continued to stand up for her beliefs both as a Weight Watchers leader and as a board member in the PTA.

Through the weight-loss process, Maggie gained lots of valuable insights into herself. And while she continues to remind herself of those lessons, she also puts them to good use in her current life, using them to continue the momentum of her success and personal growth. "The most important thing I had to learn was to be human, that it's okay to make mistakes," she says. "We just have to keep facing our challenges *and we have to continuously acknowledge our successes by pointing out to ourselves or to a friend or a loved one that it was hard but we did it. It's important because it's in that sense of triumph or success that you're going to refuel for the next time you have to do it."*

THE WELL-OILED WHEELS of the reinvention process are in motion. They're turning and turning—and you've probably begun to enjoy the ride. That's because you have all the ideas and strategies you need to go as far as you desire. At this point, the possibilities are nearly endless. And that's your own doing, a result of having given careful thought to what kind of person you want to be, to how you want to lead your life and to what your values are. By claiming responsibility for your life and by being willing to be accountable for the changes you've launched, you've put yourself in the driver's seat for the grand adventure of life, and for that you should give yourself credit. *Lots of credit.*

Each of the elements you've been cultivating for your life exerts a synergistic force on the others. Your motivation is probably strong, for example, largely because you have fully immersed yourself in the newfound sense of meaning or purpose you've embraced for your life. Your proactive approach to your goals is likely fueled by the fact that you have consciously worked so hard to shed the self-defeating beliefs that once clung to you like a stained, tattered shirt. Your performance and momentum in everyday life are likely taking a turn for the better now that you've evicted your inner critic and persuaded that winning personal coach to take up residence inside your head. Your dreams probably seem so much more doable than you'd ever imagined, simply because you've taken the time to chart a course to reach them with specific steps. And by making yourself accountable for your progress toward your goals, you're increasing your commitment to your mission—and the odds that you'll succeed.

Of course, achieving your goals can be its own reward, but you can also garner other prizes as a natural result of the self-improvement process. When you continue striving for meaningful objectives that are in sync with your personal values, when you're willing to keep moving out of your comfort zone (and, hence, expanding it), and when you're able to take charge of your time and your daily life, you'll likely gain a sense of inner peace and harmony. Your self-confidence will probably increase, your definition of yourself will broaden, you'll feel as though you have the will and the way (aka self-efficacy) to attain what you want in life, and you'll begin to understand yourself better than you used to. And hopefully you'll begin to like the person you're becoming, and begin to treat yourself as a first-class citizen by making yourself a priority and extending the same tender, loving care toward yourself that you do toward others. Then you will have truly reinvented yourself on the inside, which is where it counts the most.

Living in Harmony

Creating a more rewarding inner life is no small feat. It takes hard work and persistence. After all, you are transforming yourself from the inside out—by tapping into your central values, by taking a proactive approach to life, by examining (and correcting, when necessary) your beliefs and by improving the way you talk to yourself in your head. You've probably clarified your values and what gives your life a sense of meaning or purpose. And when you create a life that's in sync with those values, you can gain a profound sense of inner calm, a feeling of being centered in yourself and grounded in this world.

This feeling of well-being has resulted largely because you've begun to lead an integrated life, one in which all the key pieces work together, rather than against each other. When you live a more holistic life, you use your time and energy more effectively. You create a sense of balance in your life—between work and play, between action and contemplation, between giving and receiving, between being future-oriented and focused on the present. This balance helps buffer you against life's blows. If one area of your life isn't going well, you are able to turn to other areas for sustenance and support because you have carved out a rich, meaningful existence.

Indeed, by performing the soul-searching exercises in this book, you have probably developed an entirely new vision for your life. And that's wonderful! So many people travel through life blind to their secret ambitions or the dreams that would bring them peace, satisfaction and fulfillment. It may be that they're so caught up in the hurly-burly of a hectic life that they're unaware of what's most precious to them. Maybe they're so directed by what they feel they *should* do that the verb *want* is conspicuously absent from their vocabularies. Or they're afraid to recognize what they truly desire in life, especially if it's incompatible with the current state of affairs; after all, that might force them to make some unpleasant choices.

In any case, you've escaped all of these traps—and for that you should be congratulated. They say that change is the only constant in life, and while that may be true, it doesn't mean that you can't direct those changes—or at least how you respond to them. Keep reminding yourself of that because it's this truism that will allow you to create the life that you crave.

Meeting Yourself Anew

This is as good a time as any to take a brief time-out to assess how far you've come. Chances are, in the process of striving for self-improvement, you've discovered aspects of yourself that you really, really like, facets that were previously hidden under the cloak of unhappiness or unexamined behavior. Spend a few minutes thinking about how you see yourself now and jot down five positive things you've learned about yourself in the process of pursuing your goals and reading this book.

Now that you've identified these qualities and characteristics, begin to count on them as inner resources. Allow them to help you maximize your potential and become the best you that you can possibly be. You won't regret it. In fact, in a recent study involving 383 middle-aged participants, researchers at the University of Texas at Austin found that those who felt they'd lived up to their abilities scored higher in measures of overall life satisfaction. What's more, these fulfillers of self-promise were less likely to even consider going back and making different choices in the realms of work or family life, if given the opportunity, three decades later. What

Are You Taking Good Care of Yourself?

It's a good idea, now and then, to evaluate whether you're continuing to treat yourself as a top priority by taking good care of yourself physically, emotionally, mentally and spiritually. If you are, you'll be fueling your own self-discovery and self-growth processes through your actions. If you aren't, you could be draining yourself of the resources you require to continue the journey. Find out how you're doing in the self-care department by reviewing this checklist periodically:

- I am setting limits with people and requests that have the potential to drain my energy.
- I carve out personal time for myself at least once a week.
- My schedule reflects my true priorities.
- I now make conscious decisions after fully assessing the situation.
- I try to strike a balance between pursuing my goals with energy and enthusiasm and taking time to replenish my reserves with the rest and relaxation I need.
- I maintain a clear sense of who and how I want to be.
- I make an effort to appreciate my progress in various aspects of life.
- I try to let my goals and values drive my actions.
- I provide myself with a clear roadmap for how to reach my goals.
- I try to free my mind from having to remember mundane details so that it can focus on creative or intuitive pursuits.

If some of these statements turn out to be untrue for you, you'll immediately know what areas you need to work on. Your ability to stick with these principles will be tested again and again by the demands of modern life. As always, it's up to you—and only you—to see that your life reflects what truly matters most to you.

could be more phenomenal than living up to your potential, feeling content with the choices you've made and remaining highly satisfied with life, decade after decade?

In order to make the most of your potential, though, you'll need to give yourself permission to soar. This may sound obvious, but many people neglect to do just that. It's important to make a conscious decision to allow yourself to discover what drives you in life, to build on your natural talents and to bring out the qualities that make you special. And it's important to renew that commitment periodically. Think of it as akin to repledging your wedding vows—only, in this case, you're promising to continue to love, honor and treat yourself right forevermore. After all, you owe it to yourself.

Scrutinizing Your Successes

As you continue your quest to become the best you, don't ignore your teachers from the past. By now, you probably realize that mistakes present valuable learning opportunities. As the English-born actress Joan Collins once said, "Show me a person who has never made a mistake and I'll show you somebody who has never achieved much." It's wise to review your slip-ups and errors, to pull them apart, examine them from different angles and figure out what went wrong and what you can do to prevent history from repeating itself in the future.

Just as past mistakes hold useful lessons for the future, so do previous successes. If you take the time to study your successes, you can figure out what it was about your behavior or attitude that may have led to the desired outcome. What did you do right? How did your demeanor influence the situation? Once you've identified these positive elements, you can try to repeat them—altering them somewhat to suit the context of future situations, of course, but trying to reproduce what works for you. After all, you can't argue with history.

And don't forget to let yourself enjoy the successes you've been working so hard to achieve. Many people leap from one set of goals to another, as soon as they've accomplished the first, without taking time to recognize or fully digest what they've done. Or they simply attribute their success to external factors, perhaps because they're uncomfortable truly accepting their wins. It's important to take time to acknowledge how far you've come and to relish the changes. Otherwise, you could wind up undermining your commitment, self-confidence or motivation to continue striving for excellence. And you'll be depriving yourself of a sense of inherent satisfaction and meaning in what you're doing. You might celebrate these victories by treating yourself with a luxury you've been craving—a day to yourself, a particular gift, a meal at a special restaurant, whatever strikes your fancy. Most of all, it's important to allow yourself to enjoy the renewed you that's emerging from your brave actions.

Developing Your Winning Ways

One of the keys to performing at your personal best in any endeavor is to have a vivid sense of what you want. You'll want to be able to see it in your mind's eye and feel it in your heart. When you can continuously envision what you want this clearly, it's easier to go after it with passion and purpose because the desire is so well defined in your mind. With your eyes on the prize, the next step is to develop a cogent strategy for obtaining it—a strategy that includes stepping-stones that will bring you to specific goals, a time frame in which to meet them and ways to measure progress along the way. Then, you'll be ready to swing into action with gusto.

But even the best-laid plans can go awry, which is why it's important to cultivate a flexible attitude and patience. When one tactic doesn't reap the results you'd hoped for, you'll need to be willing to try another approach. When the tried-and-true measures don't come through, you'll need to be willing to take smart, calculated risks that will bring you out of your comfort zone. There's no question that this is a winning attitude that will stand you in good stead throughout your life.

Be careful, though, not to defer your happiness until some day in the distant future when the goals you're currently striving for have become a past accomplishment. As the great Russian novelist Leo Tolstoy once wrote, "If you want to be happy, be." Be yourself. Be your best. Be present in your life. And be mindful by becoming fully attentive to what you are experiencing now.

There's a reason why you are where you are in your life. You may not like the reason; it may even be unfair. But you are at this point because it's a rest stop or a roadblock along the path of *your* life. And that means you won't be able to go somewhere else until you deal with what's happening where you are right now. So you might as well try to enjoy where you are and make the most of it because this moment will never come again. And unless you're inclined to be present-minded, to focus on what you can do today that's in sync with your guiding values or mission, you may not like where you are tomorrow much better. After all, being mindfully aware of the various options at your disposal gives you greater control, according to Ellen J. Langer, Ph.D., a professor of psychology at Harvard University. And gaining a feeling of control over your life can encourage you to be more mindful. The combination can be a potent fuel for your momentum.

The Cascade of Reinvention

Personal transformation takes time; it's an ongoing process without a clear beginning or end. It's not as though the kitchen timer will ring and you'll turn out the way you want to and then the process is over. On the contrary, you may be surprised to discover that after you've embarked on the process of self-improvement and you've begun to enjoy the fruits of your efforts, you may be tempted to make more meaningful changes in your life, to enhance yourself even more by striving for new challenges.

This is a natural result of making the journey to positive change. It's rather like a beneficial domino effect: Once you begin to appreciate how possible, even probable, it is to tackle certain challenges, it seems only natural to want to take on another one, and before you know it, each positive step will help you re-create yourself or your life once more. It may be on a large scale or a small one, but the changes do add up. Pretty soon, you'll

How to Stay Body Aware

Many women have ambivalent feelings about their bodies. But the truth is, no matter what shape it's in, your body is your friend, not your enemy, and it should be treated as such. Not only is your body the home in which you live and your sole means of transportation, but it can also give you valuable clues about what's happening around you—or how you feel about it.

The key is to be willing to examine these clues. For example, sometimes physical feelings of uneasiness can be misinterpreted for hunger (the old it's-just-low-blood-sugar theory) when, in fact, those sensations could be alerting you to signs of danger or that you're feeling anxious about what's going on in a given situation. Similarly, it's often easier to blame a poor body image as a source of insecurities than to admit that you feel unsteady about your whole self. In that case, you're simply using your body as a scapegoat.

That's why it's important to stay in tune with how you feel in your body and to maintain a healthy but not obsessive awareness of your physical self. The solution is to nurture your body with healthy fuel (in the form of food, water and movement) and adequate rest and relaxation. In addition, you can befriend your body with the following strategies:

* **Conduct periodic body scans throughout the day.** Stop what you are doing for a few moments, close your eyes and mentally scan your body for signs of tension. Breathe deeply and note where the muscle kinks are or where energy doesn't seem to be flowing as fluidly as it should. This gives you the opportunity to explore sensations in your body that you wouldn't normally pay attention to. As you discover tensions and uncomfortable feel-

continued on next page

ings in various parts of your body, breathe deeply and consciously try to release that tension or discomfort from that region.

- **Unleash emotional experiences from your body.** To do this, it may help to write about the roots of your feelings about your body or to explore the underpinnings of situations where you seem to lapse into body bashing. Consider what the basis might be for feeling shame about your body. Where did it come from? What were your family's attitudes about your body or their own bodies? What is it about a particular situation that brings these feelings to the surface? You might just hit upon an event or an attitude in your life that has influenced your relationship with your body.

- **Pay attention to the thoughts and feelings that arise when you eat—or don't.** It could be that you've been using your eating habits to fill an emotional void inside you. By tuning in to how you feel when you do eat—or when you don't let yourself eat simply for emotional or stress-related reasons—you might just discover some unresolved emotional issues that are buried deep inside you. In which case, you should deal with those issues.

- **Let your personal coach check you out in the mirror.** What she sees may be far different from what you see with your own self-critical eyes. Let that benevolent inner voice point out your most attractive features or what makes you physically strong or striking. The aim is to begin to see yourself in a better, more realistic light.

- **Force yourself to face situations that produce body anxiety.** This is called desensitization, and it does work. The idea is to gradually confront the circumstances that make you physically uncomfortable, whether it's going to the gym or eating in public. It may help to start by going to low-risk situations—where you don't know anyone—then, as your comfort

continued on next page

quotient rises, to try to tackle bigger ones. By doing this, you'll slowly but surely overcome body anxiety.

- **Nurture your body's health.** If you concentrate on leading a healthier lifestyle and treating your body with the love, care and respect it deserves, you'll reclaim ownership of it. Just as you can't count on anyone else to change your life for you, it's up to you to do the best things possible for your body. It's an investment that's well worth making.

be acting like a magnet pulling good things toward yourself, attracting good fortune, new opportunities, and upbeat people in your direction. And it shouldn't be any other way.

It's healthy to keep imagining the possibilities for your life, and to welcome them with open arms. The truth is, the process of change never truly ends; you simply proceed from one cycle to another, and you keep growing in the process. After all, who you are today may be somewhat different from the way you'd like to be years from now. Your concept of the ideal you will evolve and change shape as you gain more wisdom and experience in life. Continue to use your unfolding image of the person you most want to be to help you frame goals, spur you into action, assist you in making decisions, and maintain motivation for embracing meaningful pursuits in your life. But, once again, use it flexibly. Be sure to allow yourself plenty of breathing room and ways in which to grow that your image of your ideal self may not incorporate yet.

The steps outlined in this book amount to a quality-of-life insurance plan. This is how happiness and vitality are born, how life becomes gratifying and meaningful, how people begin to fully appreciate themselves for who they are and who they can become. Whenever you find yourself being led astray or feeling overwhelmed by life's circumstances, or whenever you feel a crisis of confidence or conscience brewing, refer back to these pages. They'll help you get back in touch with what you need to do to return to the path you want to be on.

After all, this is really about designing your life the way you want it to be—and redesigning it again and again, when the urge or need strikes—rather than allowing it to be shaped by random circumstances or external forces. It's about steering the wheel as you continue the journey of your life, instead of allowing yourself to be buffeted by the winds of change. The secret to happiness is right inside you. It has been all along, and it always will be. It was just a matter of time until you were willing to dig deep enough to uncover it. Now that you've done that, you can be on your way to a life of fulfillment. It's your turn to drive. It's your turn to thrive. Nothing is preventing you from loving the life you live—or living the life you love.

ASSIGNMENT It's time to fess up one last time. How many times in your life have you said, "Someday, when I have the time, I'd like to . . ."? Since you now know that there's no such thing as free time, that you have to create the time to pursue the activities you desire, think about how you'd complete that sentence today. Home in on other activities you're interested in. What new experiences do you want to try? To get the ideas flowing, make a list from A to Z of things you'd like to try soon as well as someday in the distant future. Vow to treat yourself to one of these experiences within the next month or two. By continuing to explore new interests, you'll ward off inertia and stay in touch with your personal wish list. And that, in turn, will help you keep growing and growing . . .

CHAPTER TEN

Lessons from the Leaders

With successful weight loss under their belts, along with a variety of other accomplishments, Weight Watchers leaders have figured out more than a thing or two about what's important in life and how to achieve their dreams. They've done this by discovering the strategies that work best for them in their lives and by not being afraid to use them. Here, they offer their words of wisdom, which are based on the knowledge and perspective they've gained in the process of losing weight and striving for self-improvement.

Consider them lessons for life: The value of these little nuggets extends far beyond weight management and applies to nearly every aspect of a person's life. Feel free to borrow or steal their strategies—the leaders wouldn't have it any other way.

"Dare to ask the clarifying, crystallizing question."

What do you really want? "If you learn to ask it and answer it honestly," says Maggie Jerchau, 40, a Weight Watchers leader and trainer in Long Island, New York, "the answers and the success will follow. You have to focus on your heart because that's where all the answers are." After all, only you know what your true desires are and what will instill your life with a sense of meaning and purpose; if you can distill these values into a philosophy of life, it can serve as a mission statement that will guide you in striving for your goals.

"If you want to change your ways, do it for yourself and no one else."

That's the best recipe for success when it comes to losing weight, quitting smoking, getting fit or making any other lifestyle change. "If you do it for a loved one or an event, that's temporary," notes Sherry Fischer, 47, a Weight Watchers leader in Kentucky. "There is a beginning and an end to it. When you do it for yourself, there isn't a beginning or an end. It fits into who you are." And that difference increases the odds that the changes will become permanent because you'll be willing to do what it takes to make them that way.

"Don't wait for motivation to arrive."

"Motivation is not something that comes to you," Maggie Jerchau says. "It's something you have to seek. And the only way to find it is to take action. If you can do one thing to take control and you follow through on it, success will follow because that gives you the motivation to do more." Indeed, success does seem to breed success. When you strive for a particular goal because it's personally meaningful, you might feel energized by the changes you're making. And you might gain a sense of physical and emotional vitality, which can spur you on to continue persevering.

"Make a contract with yourself."

It doesn't have to be in legalese but it's a good idea to formalize your plans in writing. "Write down your goals and dreams and the steps you will take to achieve them," advises Jean Krueger, 56, a Weight Watchers ambassador and group leader in southern California. "Write down why you think you can do it. By writing, you can see more clearly what was only spaghetti in your head." Indeed, putting pen to paper helps clarify all sorts of goals, and it helps you commit to them because you've put them in writing.

"If something is worth doing, it's worth doing well."

Time and energy are finite, precious commodities. And there just aren't enough hours in a day or days in a week for many women to fulfill all the commitments they take on. So rather than doing a half-baked job—and depleting your time and energy in the process—make a concerted effort to stop overcommitting yourself and taking on projects that don't really matter to you. "Try to filter out what's important and what's not," says Michelle Seymour, 41, a Weight Watchers leader in New Jersey. "If something is worth pursuing, make it a priority and give it your all. If it's not worth your time and energy, let it go and move on."

"Aim to lead a conscious life."

Operating on automatic pilot can take you to exactly where you don't want to go. The trouble is, you won't even realize this until you've arrived. On the other hand, putting yourself back in the driver's seat can steer you to your desired destination. Why? Because "living mindfully helps you stay aware of your goals and dreams," notes Jenn Thomas, 28, a Weight Watchers leader in New York. "It makes you realize that you need to take small, action steps to reach your goals instead of going for instant gratification."

"Discover the strength and wherewithal inside you."

So many people can do so many things in their lives—they may be successful lawyers or stockbrokers or policemen—but they can't control their weight, notes Sharon Riguzzi, 48, a Weight Watchers leader in New York and training manager for the eastern region. "And they start beating themselves up for being weak. Weight Watchers has taught me that I'm giving them the tools. It's almost like Dorothy in *The Wizard of Oz*. They have the tools inside them; they just don't know that they're there or how to use them." Once you look inside yourself and tune into your strengths, try putting them to use in multiple areas of your life. The results may just surprise you.

"Don't be afraid to ask for support."

Changing your life doesn't have to be a solo effort. Yes, the motivation and the game plan need to come from you, if you want to achieve long-term success. But that doesn't mean you can't ask others for assistance or encouragement. Remember: "No one knows you need help unless you ask for it," Jean Krueger says. So ask trusted friends, family members, and colleagues for their support—and be specific in telling them what forms of support would help you most.

"It's important to try to see the small beauty in things."

When setting goals or striving for change, it's important to keep the big picture in mind, but not at the expense of the small details that could also be rewarding. "If you want to lose 30 pounds, even one pound is great," Thomas says. "Try to enjoy what you have and what you've done instead of always waiting for what you don't have. Yes, there's always room for improvement, but it's also important to be grateful for the small things you have and the small rewards you've earned. You don't need a fancy car to be happy; you just need four wheels."

"Strive for accountability, responsibility and consistency."

These are really the nuts and bolts of what it takes to alter your behavior permanently. Some of the biggest obstacles to change are in a person's mind-set, Seymour notes, because they're not willing to do what it takes to change. "There needs to be consistency in how you conduct your business day in and day out," she says. "And you have to be willing to take the necessary small steps to get from where you are to where you want to be." After all, nobody else can do it for you.

"Don't rush the process of change."

People often think they've changed their ways long before the behavior shifts have gelled, then they're surprised when they lapse back into their old habits. Instead of concerning yourself with a finite time frame, try to be patient and let change unfold naturally, as you concentrate your efforts on taking all the right steps. "Habits take time to change," says Sharon Walls, 42, a Weight Watchers leader in southern California. "Showing up at a Weight Watchers meeting is 95 percent of success because you're probably soaking it up without realizing it. Each week you're learning something different and that accumulation of knowledge becomes a part of you and that's what makes you successful."

"Spend time with people who have positive outlooks."

Revamping your life is hard enough without having naysayers chime in. What you need most when you're embarking on the process of change is the support and encouragement of people who are upbeat. "Winners seek out other winners," Jean Krueger says. "So seek positive people who make you feel good about yourself, not those who zap your energy and make you feel bad." You don't have to cut out the downbeat folks in your life entirely; you may just want to limit your contact with them while you're striving for your goals. If you spend your time with active, optimistic people instead, their good vibrations are likely to rub off on you.

"There's no failure until you stop trying."

Whether your goal is to slim down, run a marathon or achieve a job promotion, you can succeed if you try hard enough and stop putting unrealistic time pressures on yourself. The key is to strive for consistency and perseverance, even in the face of setbacks (which happen to everyone). Mistakes aren't anything to be ashamed of; the key is to pick yourself right up and learn from them. "It's a lot like playing sports," says Andrea Nishan, 49, a Weight Watchers leader in Massachusetts. "You may not win every game but you can still win the season. Don't be afraid to fall down; just get up when you do."

"Ease up on your expectations of yourself."

When things don't work out the way you'd hoped or you simply fall off your plan of action, it's pointless to blame or berate yourself. "It's better to say, 'Oh, well,' and forgive yourself," says Lucy Lonning, 45, a Weight Watchers leader in Connecticut. "It makes your life so much easier when you realize you don't have to be 100 percent all the time." Indeed, it's wise to do away with perfectionistic thinking and begin to hold yourself to reasonable standards, just as you would a friend. Besides, when you get to be perfect at something, you're going to be perfect at blowing it, Sharon Riguzzi adds, "because you're not going to know what to do when you make a mistake."

"It's okay to be your best friend."

Most women take better care of everyone else in their lives than they do themselves. "Everyone benefits if you take time for yourself and do things for yourself," Andrea Nishan says. Why? Because being a friend to yourself can give you more energy and enthusiasm for life, and it can boost your mood and your sense that life is meaningful and manageable. And because all of these benefits trickle down to everyone else in your life, taking care of yourself becomes a winning proposition any way you look at it. So send the guilt packing and treat yourself with the kindness and consideration that you deserve. Your whole life will profit from your friendship.

"Schedule time for yourself."

Carving out time for yourself, whether it's to exercise, relax or pursue other activities you enjoy, isn't selfish, it's smart, says Carol Immenschuh, 43, a mother of two and a Weight Watchers leader in Kansas City, Missouri, who lost 50 pounds in 1997. "You need to think about what's really important to you and about what you need to do to make your life work for you. Then you need to learn to work around the time you've set for yourself. This is time to recharge and feel better about yourself." And you should treat it as sacred. After all, when you feel good about yourself, the quality of your presence is that much better for those around you. Plus, "taking time for myself makes me a better role model for my daughters," Immenschuh adds.

"Recognize that there's no temporary fix."

On the contrary, pursuing meaningful goals is an ongoing journey, one that involves making continuous changes. "It often takes a lifelong effort to work at these goals, to practice making better choices and creating a lifestyle of healthier living, in every way possible," Immenschuh says. "You need to continue to reevaluate what's working and what's not. It helps to do a week in review, taking stock of what you did this week and whether you made yourself a priority." That way, you'll be able to pinpoint how you can fine-tune your approach for next week.

"Reward yourself for reaching milestones along the way to your goal."

When striving for goals, it's smart to make them specific in terms of the results you want to achieve but then to break each one up into small, manageable pieces. This way, the pursuit becomes much less daunting. While you're at it, "attach tangible rewards to meeting those milestones," advises Dawn Young, 37, a Weight Watchers leader in Fountain, Colorado, who lost 34 pounds in 1992. "The reward makes it more fun and it serves as a reminder that you've succeeded. Success breeds success."

"If you tell yourself something often enough, you will come to believe it."

So you might as well talk kindly to yourself and try to cultivate a positive attitude. "Tell yourself that you can reach your goal; read books or stories about people who have overcome challenges; write positive notes to yourself and post them around your home," Young suggests. "It's 100 times easier to reach your goals if you have a positive attitude." Why? Because you'll be acting as your own coach and cheerleader, bolstering your resolve and energy along the way, instead of working against yourself, as you would if your mind-set were negative. With a positive attitude, "gradually, you'll come to believe that you really can do this," Young adds, "and then it will happen."

"It's important to start somewhere."

"Sometimes you start with a goal in mind and as you proceed, more and more opportunities present themselves just because you've started," explains Angela Barnett, 38, a Weight Watchers leader in Minneapolis who lost 50 pounds in 1995. "Making the choice to begin sets the wheels in motion and that makes so many other things possible. That awareness lightbulb goes on and you start to become aware of all sorts of opportunities that might have been there all along." By making one small change, you put yourself in a position to be ready to take the next step and take advantage of new opportunities that come your way.

"The more you do, the more you'll want to do."
As you begin to make small but meaningful changes in your life, you'll start to realize how truly possible some of your other aspirations are. "Once you realize you can do it, you're more willing to take risks because you feel more capable," Barnett says. "And it's because you're gaining confidence. Then you might start doing a little bit more and a little bit more . . . and before you know it, you're accomplishing things you didn't know were possible for you." That's one of the hidden gifts that comes with successfully changing a part of your life.

Recommended Reading

Benson, Herbert, and Eileen Stuart. *The Wellness Book: The Comprehensive Guide to Maintaining Health and Treating Stress-Related Illness*. New York: Fireside, 1992.

Brandt, David. *Is That ALL There Is? Balancing Expectation and Disappointment in Your Life*. San Luis Obispo, Calif.: Impact, 1998.

Burns, David D. *The Feeling Good Handbook*. New York: Plume, 1999.

Cash, Thomas. *What Do You See When You Look in the Mirror? Helping Yourself to a Positive Body Image*. New York: Bantam, 1995.

Csikszentmihalyi, Mihaly. *Flow: The Psychology of Optimal Experience*. New York: HarperCollins, 1990.

Deci, Edward, with Richard Flaste. *Why We Do What We Do: The Dynamics of Personal Autonomy*. New York: G.P. Putnam's Sons, 1995.

Domar, Alice, and Henry Dreher. *Self-Nurture: Learning to Care for Yourself as Effectively as You Care for Everyone Else*. New York: Viking, 2000.

Langer, Ellen J. *Mindfulness*. Reading, Mass.: Perseus, 1989.

Murphy, Shane. *The Achievement Zone: 8 Skills for Winning All the Time from the Playing Field to the Boardroom*. New York: G. P. Putnam's Sons, 1996.

Myers, David. *The Pursuit of Happiness: Discovering the Pathway to Fulfillment, Well-being, and Enduring Personal Joy*. New York: Avon, 1992.

Prochaska, James, John Norcross, and Carlo DiClemente. *Changing for Good: The Revolutionary Program that Explains the Six Stages of Change and Teaches You How to Free Yourself from Bad Habits.* New York: Morrow, 1994.

Williams, Virginia, and Redford Williams. *Lifeskills.* New York: Times Books, 1997.

Index

"thin" attitude, 108
thinking ahead, 74
Thomas, Jenn, 106–9, 205, 206
Thoreau, Henry David, 62
thoughts, in tune with, 116–17
time, for yourself, 208
time log, 141
time management, 57, 74, 141–43, 204
timing:
    importance of, 68, 69, 70–71
    seizing the moment in, 75
    success and, 66–68
to do list, 61–62
Tolstoy, Leo, 198
transformation, 198–202
trend tracking, 99–100
trigger factors, 86, 140
truth, living in, 11–12

vacation from worries, 170
victim, thinking like, 16–17
viewpoints, new, 179–80
vigor, mental, 75, 122–23, 165
visualization:
    of control, 140
    of excellence, 91
    of new ideas, 178
    of the possibilities, 46–48, 49, 201
    of relaxation, 158, 166
    of success, 164
    of your goals, 197–98
    see also dreams
vitality, subjective, 54

Walls, Sharon, 15–18, 206–7
weak spots, handling of, 164
weight gain:
    causes of, 15
    eating habits and, 190

pregnancy and, 129
triggers of, 86, 140
weight loss:
    as catalyst for other changes, 44
    contract for, 67–68
    dieting as only one factor in, 15–16
    energy level and, 89
    insights into self via, 191
    physical activity and, 17–18, 42, 43–44,
        106–7, 129–30, 150–51, 190
    plateau in, 174–75, 176–77
    regaining, 172
    reinvention via, 12
    self-confidence and, 130
    successful dieters at, 171
    in Weight Watchers, see Weight Watchers
        stories
Weight Watchers:
    on change, 169
    lessons from, 203–10
    positive influence of, 12, 16–18, 43,
        66–68, 87–89, 107–9, 128–30,
        150–51, 172–74, 189–91
Weight Watchers stories:
    Fischer, 65, 66–68
    Jerchau, 187–92
    Krueger, 41–45
    Lonning, 148–52
    Nishan, 85–86, 87–89
    Riguzzi, 127, 128–30
    Seymour, 169, 171, 172–74
    Thomas, 106–9
    Walls, 15–18
well-being, 19–20, 53, 193
winners, seeking, 207
workplace, stressful, 135–36, 177
worries, vacation from, 170

Young, Dawn, 209

Credits for Photo Insert